Maggie Jones writes on health and pend-
ent, the *Guardian* and the *Obs* She is also a qualified
breast-feeding counsellor for the National Childbirth Trust. Her
original research on the subjects of cystitis and thrush has
unearthed much new information which dispels the widely
accepted myths about these and other infections in this area. She
worked for the Family Planning Association for five years and
has travelled for the WHO and IPPF.

Maggie is married with three children and lives in East London.

Jacky Fleming is a best-selling cartoonist. Her latest book,
Falling in Love was published by Penguin.

Line drawings by **Noel Chamberlain**.

BELOW THE BELT

Self help for cystitis and thrush

Maggie Jones

HEADLINE

First published in 1995
by HEADLINE BOOK PUBLISHING

10 9 8 7 6 5 4 3 2 1

ISBN 0 7472 4706 4

Typeset by
Letterpart Limited, Reigate, Surrey

Printed and bound in Great Britain by
Cox & Wyman Ltd, Reading, Berkshire

HEADLINE BOOK PUBLISHING
A division of Hodder Headline PLC
338 Euston Road
London NW1 3BH

Contents

Acknowledgements

I am extremely grateful to Dr Angela Robinson, consultant physician at the Mortimer Market Centre Sexual Health Clinic, for scrupulously checking the facts in this book.

Introduction

Thrush and cystitis are two of the most common complaints experienced by women. As many as four out of five women will have an attack of cystitis at some time in their lives and about three-quarters of women will experience thrush at some point too. Yet these complaints are not much talked about and women remain in ignorance about their symptoms, causes and cures, mainly because they are considered just 'not nice'.

Newspapers and magazines, while full of information on other illnesses and problems which affect women, tend to keep quiet about these complaints too. Let's face it, there's nothing very 'sexy', as journalists say, about these topics. Indeed, the very opposite, because one of the most distressing aspects of thrush and cystitis for many women is that they make sex painful, difficult or even impossible. And to make matters worse, episodes of thrush and cystitis can often be triggered by sex.

Because many women don't know what causes thrush and cystitis, they are afraid that doctors and others will think that they don't keep themselves clean, or that they've been sleeping around. A recent survey carried out by Gallup Poll showed that almost one in five women wrongly thought that thrush was caused by poor hygiene and that one in ten thought that it was due to promiscuous behaviour. Some women mistake the symptoms of both thrush and cystitis for a sexually transmitted disease.

Depression too can be a feature of cystitis and thrush for many women. The feeling of never being well, of never being able to enjoy life, of having to avoid sex, certain foods, take drugs, and face the endless cycle of visits backwards and forwards to the doctor's surgery, all take their toll. It's not surprising that many women get deeply depressed and sometimes even have suicidal thoughts. The stresses in your relationship too can lead to depression, especially if it looks like it is breaking down completely. Just knowing that this is normal and that other sufferers feel depressed can help you put this in perspective; you are not alone!

What exactly are cystitis and thrush?

CYSTITIS

Cystitis is an infection or inflammation of the bladder and the tube which carries urine from the bladder to the outside, known as the urethra. It comes from two Latin words, 'cyst' meaning pouch or sac, and 'itis' meaning inflammation. Its symptoms are:

★ Burning or pain during urination (peeing)
★ An urgent need to urinate
★ Frequent urge to urinate
★ Frequent waking at night to urinate
★ Pain above the pelvic bone and lower back
★ Blood-tinged urine

Typically its symptoms start with a need to pee frequently, and often the urine stings. As the attack gets worse, the symptoms can be intolerable, with the sensation that you want to pee all the time, and sometimes can't stop yourself either. The pain can be excruciating – one woman described it as 'peeing broken glass'. In a severe attack there is often blood

2

in the urine and the whole abdominal area can feel sore and uncomfortable. Women often also run a temperature.

Cystitis can be serious – if left untreated, the infection can ascend up the tubes called ureters to the kidneys. A kidney infection usually results in fever, shivering, and pain in the kidney area. Untreated, this can lead to damage of the kidneys which can be serious. So cystitis should never be neglected.

Your first attack of cystitis can be frightening as well as very unpleasant. The suddenness with which it can start, the pain, the loss of control over urinating, and the sight of blood in the urine, can terrify anyone who has never heard of this condition. One woman recalls the relief she felt when she went into hospital in the middle of the night, convinced she had been stricken down with some rare and terrifying illness, to be told, 'Oh, it's only cystitis!' '*Only* cystitis!' echoes another woman, listening to this anecdote. 'Only someone who's never suffered from it could ever say that!'

The shock and misery of a first attack can be devastating. 'It was with a new boyfriend, someone I was really keen on,' recalls Alison. 'We went to bed for the first time the previous day and we made love several times. I woke up in the middle of the night with this awful pain and I spent the whole night on the loo, peeing, crying with the pain, drinking, peeing again. I didn't get a minute's sleep. I could hear the snores of my boyfriend in the next room, sleeping peacefully, completely oblivious of what I was going through. At that moment I hated him! But I didn't want to wake him and explain because it seemed so shameful. I have never felt more lonely and the pain was worse than anything I had imagined.'

If a woman has repeated attacks of cystitis the wall of the urethra may become scarred and this may make the woman prone to more attacks. So trying to deal with the condition as soon as it occurs and preventing a recurrence is very important for the future.

THRUSH

Thrush is a fungal infection which can affect the vagina and the vulva (outer lips of the vagina). Its symptoms are:

★ A sore or itchy vulva which may be mild or severe
★ Discharge from the vagina, more profuse than normal
★ Pain, swelling and redness of the vagina and vulva
★ Discomfort when anything is put into the vagina, such as a tampon or when having sex
★ Soreness and pain on passing urine

Thrush is caused by a common fungus of the yeast family called Candida albicans, which is usually present on women's skin, in their bowel and vagina, without causing any symptoms. Although it is a member of the yeast family, it is a different organism to the usual yeast that we use for baking bread and fermenting wine. If the fungus takes a hold it causes itching, redness and soreness of the vaginal area and often a white discharge can be seen, looking a little like cottage cheese. In some women the discharge can be thick and gunky, in others it's watery with little white flecks in it. The irritation of the vulval area can also lead to symptoms similar to the beginnings of an attack of cystitis, such as a desire to pee frequently and soreness as the urine stings the inflamed skin.

Although these are two separate and distinct conditions, thrush and cystitis are often linked. This is because cystitis is usually treated with antibiotics, and antibiotics often make thrush flare up. The fungus lives on most women's skin all the time, but is kept in check by the normal bacteria which also live on the skin. Thrush favours the warm, moist environment of the vagina and genitals. When antibiotics kill off these protective bacteria, thrush multiplies and invades.

On the other hand, thrush can help lead to cystitis too. The fungus provides a good breeding ground for the harmful kinds of bacteria which lead to cystitis. All too often a woman gets into a vicious circle of attacks of cystitis, followed by antibiotics, followed by thrush, followed by yet another attack of cystitis.

TAKING IT SERIOUSLY

One problem with thrush and cystitis is that until recently doctors have failed to take these really seriously. Cystitis, they think, is easily treated by antibiotics so is no more of a nuisance than a sore throat. Thrush can be treated with antifungal creams. If women come back repeatedly, doctors may go a little further and try to look at other causes and suggest some ways of avoiding repeat attacks. They often do not realise the misery and harm to women's self-image and their relationships which repeated attacks can cause.

Nora's story
Nora was twenty-seven when she met Jim at a friend's house. They started going out together and soon fell in love. After a few months Nora moved in with him and the couple assumed that they would get married.

Soon after the first time they made love, Nora had a severe attack of cystitis. The doctor prescribed antibiotics and she was soon better, although the pain of that first attack was etched in her memory. The doctor told her that 'honeymoon cystitis' was very common and that the problem shouldn't recur. Unfortunately it did, repeatedly. Nora took a lot of time off work and went to a number of different doctors to try to get help with her problem. In the meantime, she came to dread sex, and would often make excuses like feeling tired or under the weather to avoid the act which so often led to a flare-up of the dreaded cystitis. Although Jim was initially sympathetic, he didn't have to tolerate the pain and thought that cystitis could easily be treated by a day off work and a speedy visit to the doctor. He began to think that Nora was making an unnecessary fuss.

A year after moving in with Jim, Nora moved out. Their relationship was falling apart and Nora thought that if they lived separately this might reintroduce the spark. It didn't. Within a year Jim had met someone else and married her. They now have two children; Nora is still single and still suffering from cystitis.

This is far from the only relationship or even marriage which has failed because repeated attacks of cystitis and thrush have put a woman off sex. It would be nice if true love could overcome such problems, but the reality is that it often does not. As one woman said, 'It's very hard to feel sexy when your private parts itch and you've got a gunky discharge.' What's more, people often mistake or confuse cystitis and thrush for sexually transmitted diseases and have to deal with all the negative attitudes to that.

Claire made a classic error when she started a new sexual relationship after a long period on her own. A few days after making love she had a thick, itchy discharge. She wasn't sure what it was and was anxious and upset. When she saw the man that night she told him that he had 'given her an infection' and they couldn't make love, and that she was going to the GUM (Genito-urinary Medicine) clinic the next day. It turned out to be thrush and yes, the relationship was short-lived!

FINDING A CURE

Fortunately, today there is prompt and effective treatment available for both cystitis and thrush, and also for other vaginal infections. This is very different from how it was in the past, although cystitis has been recognised as a disease from early times, and old Egyptian papyri give recipes for urinary symptoms such as juniper berries, cumin and coriander. Hippocrates, the Greek doctor who lived in 500 BC and was responsible for the Hippocratic oath, made many references to urinary disorders and suggested that the urine should be closely inspected for signs of sediment, particles and pus, a practice still carried out by doctors today, albeit in a more sophisticated way.

In 1635 the famous herbalist Nicholas Culpepper advised red coral, marshmallow in goat's milk, and burnt mice in milk for urinary symptoms.

It was in 1863 that Pasteur noticed that urine made a good medium for growing bacteria, and in 1881 Roberts made the link between bacteria in the urine and symptoms of pain and frequency in urinating. In 1894 a German doctor, Escherich, was to describe a bacterium in the urine of children, and the bacterium became known as Escherichia coli. This is the most common bacterium causing urinary tract infections today.

While treatment for cystitis seems to have been relatively humane, that for thrush was sometimes barbaric. Any diseases of the reproductive organs tended to be blamed on women's inherent frailty or on signs of sexual feelings which were considered abnormal. Treatments for thrush then included deliberate blistering of the groin and thighs, the application of leeches to the genitals, and even surgical removal of the clitoris.

Although today antibiotics have revolutionised treatment for cystitis and anti-fungal agents provide a cure for thrush, a great deal of confusion still exists about the treatment of cystitis and recurrent thrush. Women often find that medical treatment is not all it should be, so try self help and alternative methods of coping with cystitis; but sometimes these treatments contradict one another. Although much research has been done, not all doctors are aware of it, and medical experts, practitioners of alternative medicine and others all have very different views, so it's not surprising that women become confused, angry and distressed.

Further, doctors very seldom realise the extent to which repeated attacks of thrush and cystitis can devastate your sex life. Women feel unclean and inadequate, and can become obsessed with hygiene. Men feel guilty that they are causing their partners such pain and both parties often retreat from sex, damaging their happiness and sometimes their relationships, as we have seen above.

Many women, fed up with the standard medical advice, turn to alternative and self-help treatments. Much of the present knowledge of self-help techniques for cystitis comes from Angela Kilmartin. When Angela Kilmartin suffered an acute attack of cystitis on her honeymoon in August 1966, she little realised how this painful condition was going to wreak havoc with her life and marriage over the following years. At the time the only medical treatment was to dish out antibiotics; no information was given on dealing with the symptoms or preventing a recurrence. Since her attacks usually came on after sex, she was twice told to stop having sex for six months, despite which she still suffered several attacks. Needless to say, this played havoc with her married life.

She had two cystoscopies – operations to view the inside of the bladder – and dilations of the urethra, followed by a cauterisation of the urethra to 'burn away the infected skin'. These did not make any difference to her condition; in fact, they may have added to the damage caused by repeated attacks of cystitis. Six weeks after the cauterisation she had another attack and felt suicidal for the first and only time.

Finally she found a hospital consultant who told her always to get up and pee after having sex. This was the first piece of advice which seemed to help the problem; it was followed by the first three-month period in which she didn't have an attack of cystitis. Inevitably her question was, 'Why didn't anyone tell me this before? And what else do you know which might help?'

She asked for a meeting with medical staff at Bart's hospital, London, to help draft a leaflet for patients on self help, prevention and cure of cystitis. Angela Kilmartin dedicated the next twenty years of her life to making sure that other women would know about simple, self-help remedies and preventatives for cystitis so no one should have to suffer as she did. She has written six books on cystitis, appeared on numerous radio and television programmes and founded the U and I self-help group, which she ran tirelessly for ten years until it folded in 1981. One hospital consultant estimated that with her self-help techniques she alone had cut down the number of women with urinary tract infections presenting at his hospital clinic by 80%.

Despite all her work, however, and the fact that much of her advice has been quite widely adopted by doctors, recurrent cystitis can still wreak havoc with people's lives. For those who think that cystitis is a temporary or trivial complaint, the story of Kelly is a typical example of how, even today, a woman's life can be wrecked by repeated attacks of cystitis and thrush.

Kelly's story
'When I was ten, going on eleven, I had terrible cystitis. I didn't realise what it was. I just remember it being terribly painful. I had a kidney infection and they discovered that one of my kidneys was scarred. I don't know whether this kidney damage caused the cystitis or whether the cystitis caused the damage . . . When I was seventeen I had another bout, I remember being ill for five or six weeks one summer, and trying to keep my feet warm all the time because I thought it was related to getting chilled.

'The first time I slept with my current partner it happened . . . Halfway through the next day I suddenly thought, "Oh God". I knew what it was. I went to the chemist and got Cystemme or one of those over-the-counter remedies . . . that was on a Monday. I'd just started a job, it was my first day. I don't know what they thought, they must have thought I was mad because I kept on disappearing to the loo. It got a bit better but then in the night it was unbearable and I knew I was going to have to get antibiotics.

'I went to the doctor and got amoxycillin, took them for two days and carried on drinking lots of water. It cleared up and by 4–5 days I was back to normal. I wasn't too worried. I thought, well, I knew why it was – I hadn't had sex for a long time, I wasn't properly lubricated, I was in a bad temper because I knew I had to get up early in the morning and start the new job – but four weeks later the same thing happened. Again I thought I knew why it was – I'd been to see my mother and I was angry with her, I was feeling very tense. Again it quickly became very acute – I had to take antibiotics, this time trimethoprim – but by the second day it was much better and by the weekend it was back to normal.

'That was in April; in August it happened again. I didn't wait this time; I went first thing in the morning to the GP as I had to go to work. I took the same antibiotics and they worked quite quickly and even by the evening it was much better. I felt all right about it, I felt I could manage and contain the attacks. My doctor gave me antibiotics and told me to take them straight away the moment I felt the symptoms beginning, so I did this. I now wish I hadn't . . .

'A bit later it started again and I took the antibiotics. It didn't get very acute, but it seemed to drag on for about a week with slight burning when I peed, and I felt uncomfortable all the time. I took more antibiotics. When I went away on holiday it was still like that and then it became a full, rip-roaring, full-scale attack. I couldn't get off the loo for about

10

one and a half hours, peeing all the time, and it was agony. I felt almost suicidal. My temperature was 104, I was shaking. I had to walk to the chemist in the village and they said they couldn't help, I'd have to see the doctor.

'The doctor said, have you been drinking fizzy drinks? and I said, no, not particularly, nor fizzy water, but I said I had been drinking bicarbonate of soda and he told me that was very bad, and hot water bottles were bad. By then I'd read various books on cystitis so I was doing all those things, drinking a pint of water every twenty minutes, bicarbonate of soda, hot water bottle between the thighs for the pain. I was still on antibiotics and some strange liquid which turned my urine blue . . . I showed him the antibiotics and he prescribed another sort, they were French so I don't know what they were. At first the attacks had come about seven or eight hours after sex but this time I had felt a bit odd and it happened just 1–2 hours after sex.

'By now I was getting afraid of proper sex. After about 3–4 weeks we had sex, but no penetration. I had followed the books' advice and washed myself before and after, but later on that day it started. I thought if I drank lots and lots of water and sodium bicarb it would go away, but by Tuesday it was obviously not going away. The doctor gave me the same old antibiotics but took a urine sample. Within a week they rang and said, yes, you have got an infection and it's resistant to the antibiotics you've been given. My doctor said he thought these had all been the same infection, and that because it was resistant to the antibiotics all they'd done was stun it for a bit and then it had come back, and that made sense to me. I thought, now I'll get rid of it! I took the new antibiotic, nitro-furantoin, and that seemed to do the trick. That was in October.

'But in November it happened again, and I also had a discharge which I thought was thrush. At that point I started going to a homeopath because I thought I was taking far too many antibiotics and there must be an alternative. The homeopath said oh, there are lots and lots of remedies, and she started me on pulsatilla and staphysagria. What I found frustrating was that I had this burning discharge all the time, which was really uncomfortable, and in some ways it was worse than cystitis because it just went on and on and it wasn't something I could control. It was a sort of yellow, watery discharge which left yellow stains on my underwear. It was never itchy, it was only ever sore. So I tried things for that – I went onto sepia and sulphur, and I tried lots of Canesten cream, but it didn't seem to make any difference. I was trying the homeopathic remedies from November till March – I'd given up with the GP. The homeopath said, oh, they'll just give you more antibiotics which won't help, and it always gets worse before it gets better. Do nothing at all for a week and see how it settles down, see if it gets any better. I even had a massage, and I went to a friend of mine who does healing.

'The trouble with homeopathy was we seemed to spend hours talking about exact symptoms – is it stinging, is it burning? It's a funny language they use, and it all seems so imprecise. On the other hand, I was clear of actual cystitis for quite a while when seeing the homeopath, so I did think it must be working.

'Eventually when the discharge wouldn't go away I went to the GUM clinic. This was unfortunately in a week when the discharge wasn't very bad, and they said they couldn't really see a discharge; in fact it looked a bit dry, and the swabs came back negative. They asked was I using soaps etc. and I said I hadn't used any for I don't know how long. They gave me something else to use instead of soap, and that evening, because of the examination, it was dreadful, and the aqueous solution they gave me made it even worse. I went on an anti-candida diet, and then I got this really thick discharge back again. I went back to my doctor, and he couldn't be bothered to do a swab; he just prescribed Diflucan, for thrush, and it did seem to get better then.

'My GP said he thought the pain was coming from my bladder muscle, which didn't know what was going on and kept on contracting, which made me feel I'd got symptoms, so he also prescribed something called Ditropan (oxybutanin). This relaxes your bladder muscle. I took it four times a day. I hadn't had a bad attack of cystitis then from November till April. By then my friends had all labelled me a complete neurotic. They suggested I went to see a hypnotist, said I should stop thinking about it, that it ruled my life . . .

'Then I went to see a specialist at St Pancras who had a good reputation, because I was still getting pain before and after urinating. He'd told a friend that she was bringing on her symptoms herself with too much self-help treatment, drinking too many fluids, too much sodium bicarb etc., and that she didn't actually have infections. They were going to do a bladder function test but he didn't want to put a catheter in because he said my urethra was inflamed and I would just go up the wall. He measured the pH of my vagina and said it was alkaline. He thought I'd got anaerobic vaginosis, and that this might not have shown up on the swab at the GUM clinic, and he prescribed Flagyl. I started taking those and then that night the cystitis started. I rang him and he said he thought I'd got a bladder infection and prescribed Macrodantin. I brought in a specimen and the result came back and he said no, there wasn't an infection, he thought we were dealing with urethritis, possibly caused by chlamydia, but rather than take a swab, because it's hard to trace, and because I was sore, why not use hydrocortisone cream. I said my hydrocortisone cream said all over it, don't use on the genital area, and he laughed and said, it's all right to use it a bit, so I used it for about a week.

'Then two weeks later I had to pee a lot in the night. I tried to keep my legs apart and relax but it was excruciatingly painful. I took some cantharis, which I still had from the homeopath. Nothing happened, so I took potassium citrate. I thought, this is urethritis again. I remember wondering, I don't know how my system can get back to normal after all this. I never enjoyed myself, no alcohol because of the antibiotics, no sex.

'I woke up in the morning and I felt better, so I thought I wouldn't go and see the doctor, I'd just hand in a specimen. It looked awful first thing in the morning, but they said no, you must do one in a sterile container this afternoon, and by then it looked quite clear and normal. Then the next day it became really severe. I couldn't go out, I felt so awful, and the pain was so bad I thought, if I cut my wrists could it be worse? I felt suicidal. I felt I was falling into a deep pit, it was worse than ever. I thought maybe the cantharis had made it worse, because in homeopathic medicine if you take too much it makes it worse. It's always so non-specific – you can't stop taking it till you're better, but if you're a bit better and you stop taking it it can make you worse, so I thought, I'll just drink water and have nothing at all. I rested and the next day I felt a bit better. I carried on feeling better for two or three days, but then on the Wednesday I got the most terrific pain across my hip and back like a stitch.

'I rang the doctor and said I'd taken in a specimen the week before and he said, oh actually yes, there's a prescription for you here, Macrodantin. I said, I took that two weeks ago, I don't want to take it again, so he prescribed Septrin. I had this pain just before and after peeing, the pain in my back was worse and I had a temperature. He said that was a bit worrying in case it affected my kidneys. On Friday afternoon my temperature went down. I went for a walk and then I had to lie down. I was supposed to be going away the next day, so I drove to my boyfriend's with this really bad pain in my back and collapsed when I got there. I went to the surgery the next morning and they said take some ibuprofen (Nurofen) and double the dose of antibiotics. I said, I haven't taken my temperature but I know it's very high, I have a terrific pain in my side and I'm feeling very sick, and they repeated the advice and said come back on Tuesday. It was the Saturday of a bank holiday weekend – it always seems to happen on Saturdays. I rang my sister who is a GP and she said, don't worry, go into casualty and get an ambulance if you have to, it's your kidneys and you have to get in there. In casualty they took a specimen, about two drops; it was agony peeing.

'The good thing about being in hospital was that they could do all the tests straight away. They said there were lots of bacteria in my urine and the antibiotics I was taking weren't doing anything. The blood cell count was very high. They sent me for X-Rays and took me onto the ward, put me on a drip and gave me intravenous antibiotics and pethidine, because I was writhing by then. They had to lift me up to pee, and I was throwing up bile, which I thought was the most alarming thing, because it looked like pee. I just thought, my whole system has broken down, it's coming out of my stomach! I thought I'd be in for a day or two but in fact I was in for ten days. I thought they would find something, a kidney stone or something, which was causing all this. I thought if they could find a cause there would be something they could do to end all this misery.

'They said no, there's no kidney stone. I mentioned the kidney scars from when I was a child but they didn't seem to think that was the reason; the scan just showed the right kidney was enlarged from nine to thirteen centimetres due to the infection. They did a test at the end and said that the urine was clear, and it occurred to me that they'd never done a test at the end of treatment before to see if it was clear. I'd heard of something called cystitis cystica where there are cysts in the bladder which can harbour bacteria and wondered if this could apply to me.

'I eventually talked to the urologist and he said lots and lots of women get this problem. He told me about personal hygiene, not using soaps or scented anything, drinking lots of fluids and not getting constipated, because this can go with dehydration and also can cause stress during intercourse, so I should eat a high-fibre diet. He also told me about emptying the bladder after sex, never going too long without peeing, and all that.

'He said: "What we have to look at is the fact that you've had six known infections as well as everything else, and we have to look at treating that. Your kidneys seem to be all right, they couldn't see a stone or anything."

'They didn't test for a blockage, which might cause urine to stagnate, but they will do a flexible cystoscopy to look at the lining of the bladder, but in most women of my age there isn't anything visibly wrong. They can't do this for 4–6 weeks after an infection, so I have to wait for that.

'They said if that's all clear they'll give me a low dose of antibiotics to take every day on four-monthly cycles so I don't build up a resistance. Apparently this can help reduce the number of attacks from 6–12 attacks every year to one or two. I don't know how women cope with 6–12 attacks every year without killing themselves.

'Incidentally, after a gynaecological examination the gynae-cologist said I had a cervical ectopia. It's not a problem, but I wondered if this had caused the discharge.

'What upset me was that I left hospital without any reassurance that in a few days this just won't happen again.

'The worst thing about it is what it's done to my relation-ship. After a while sex and pain become inextricable in your mind and the whole thing becomes a terrible wedge between you. There's a lot of contention between you about who's caused what and if you're passing one another thrush and if he's caused you to be ill. I also feel it makes you feel a failure as a woman. I feel that I can't have sex, I'm not a proper woman. There's anguish, anxiety, tension, and I think it's my fault, that perhaps I tense up without realising it. But I've had attacks without having sex – that doesn't seem to be the cause any more. I've met plenty of people who say, oh I had three or four attacks when I had a new relationship and then it just stopped, but with me it's just gone on and on.

'I think there must be a weak point in your body which gives when you're under stress, and that's mine. I've read about Chinese medicine and yin and yang and all that, I tried acupuncture, but I don't know. I've tried everything. I've even tried special diets for thrush and cystitis, but trying to cope with that and any kind of normal social life is impossible, and then you become even more isolated and everyone else thinks you're neurotic – no coffee, no alcohol, no sugar. So then I got so sick of it I did have the odd drink and it didn't get any worse. At one point the homeopath said no sex, no alcohol for four weeks, you must do this or it'll just keep coming back; but I did that and it still kept coming back. And my working life has been completely torn apart. I'm a freelance researcher and my work just dwindled away because I was always getting ill.

I don't suppose you know which remedies you've tried so far?

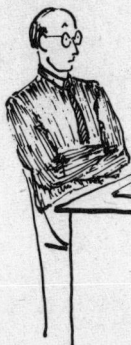

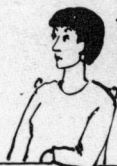

Cystemme, amoxycillin, trimethoprim, bicarbonate of soda, pulsatilla, staphysagria, Ditropan, oxybutanin, Flagyl, Macrodantin, hydrocortisone cream, Canesten, cantharis, potassium citrate, Septrin, ibuprofen, and yoghurt – live

'All I want is a reason why this keeps happening to me. If they could give me a reason and tell me they could do something to put an end to it, I could hope that there might be a cure.'

Is there hope for Kelly? Yes, there should be. The good news is that the misery of both thrush and cystitis can be alleviated or prevented with the help of a few basic precautions and treatments, which may not even involve visiting your doctor. If these don't work, then prompt medical treatment can cut short the attack and alleviate the suffering. Some changes in lifestyle and habits can make all the difference, and with any luck, banish these conditions for ever. If you're reading this book because you've suffered your first attack, let's hope it will be your last. And if you've suffered from either for years, you may find here the clue that will also help you towards a life free from the misery of thrush and cystitis.

CHAPTER 1
Cystitis

HOW YOU GET IT

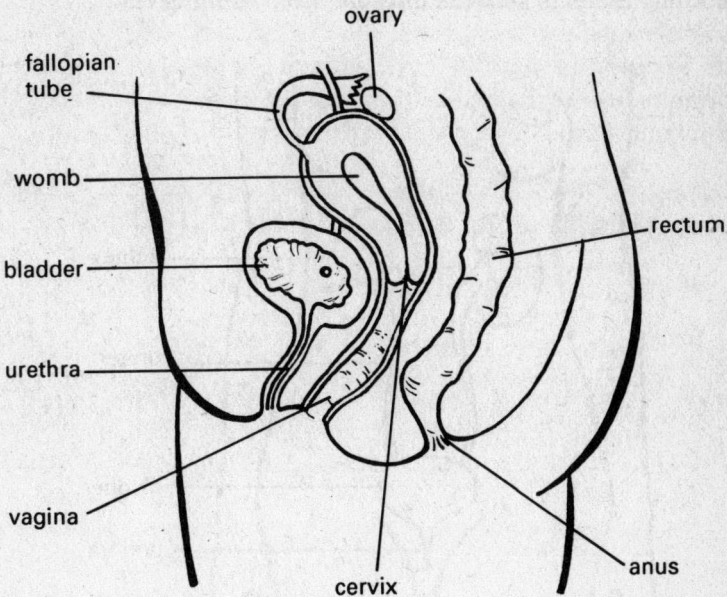

Let's admit it – the basic cause of cystitis is the poor design of
the female body, or, more precisely, its genital area. As

someone once pointed out, it was rather a mistake of the creator to place the pleasure garden in between the sewers! Bacteria – germs – from the gut are expelled at the anus and no matter how careful you are in wiping your bottom and washing your hands, some bacteria will remain on the skin. These can work their way into the urethra, the opening which leads back to the bladder and through which urine is passed, and multiply rapidly in the stored urine, leading to cystitis.

Many human secretions such as tears, saliva and catarrh contain immune substances which help kill off bacteria, but urine does not. In fact, it provides an ideal breeding ground for many bacteria. So, once bacteria get into the bladder, there is nothing much to stop the infection from running riot.

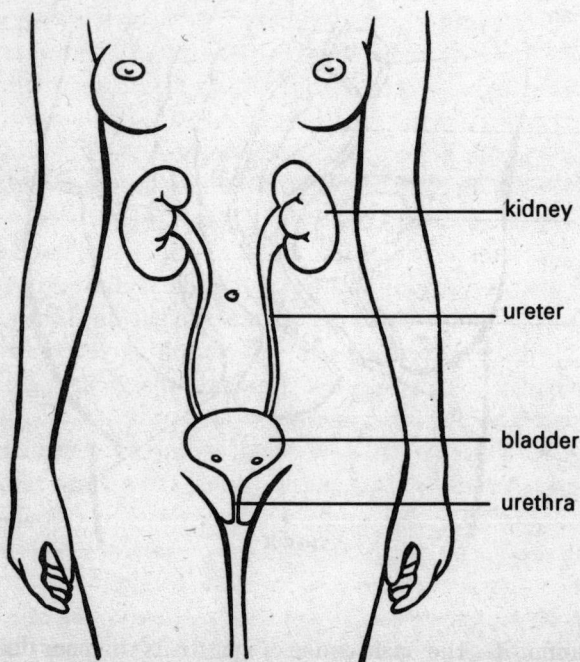

kidney

ureter

bladder

urethra

To understand cystitis, it's important to understand a little about how the urinary system works. The diagram opposite shows the kidneys, the ureters – the tubes which lead from the kidneys to the bladder – the bladder and the urethra, which carries the urine to the outside. Urine contains waste products from the body's metabolism which the body doesn't need and which would actually be toxic if left in the blood-stream. The kidneys filter out these harmful substances and tend to work at a fairly constant rate, though they tend to slow down when you are asleep and speed up when you are exercising vigorously. This is why you don't usually need to pee overnight and why you may need to pee after taking exercise. Valves at the exit from the kidneys prevent urine from passing backwards back into the kidneys.

The urine passes down the ureters into the bladder, where it is stored. When the bladder becomes full, 'stretch receptors' in the bladder wall become active and messages are sent to the brain to register this and give you the sensation of wanting to pee. Most people seem to pee when the bladder contains about half a pint, and the bladder becomes extremely uncomfortable once more than a pint has been stored.

The sphincter muscles around the neck of the bladder and another at the vaginal opening are under voluntary control, so adults can 'hang on' when they want to pee until they are in a suitable place. When you are really bursting you tend to use other muscles to constrict the opening, cross your legs, jiggle about and resort to other devices!

Small children do not yet have voluntary control of the bladder and the urine is expelled by reflex at a certain point, and some old people lose this ability too. There is often a lot of shame associated with losing control of these muscles, which can be caused by the blame inflicted on small children who are late gaining bladder control, and wet their clothes or the bed. In an attack of cystitis, inflammation of the urethra and bladder confuse the usual signals and often create the sensation of wanting to pee all the time. Some women with cystitis do lose control of the sphincter muscle and wet themselves, though usually there is not much to pee at any one time.

In women, the urethra is very short, only about one and a half inches. Compare this with the man's, which has to run the whole length of his penis! The woman's short urethra makes it much easier for germs to find their way up into the bladder, which is why cystitis is much rarer in men than it is in women. In men cystitis is often linked to kidney or prostate problems and warrants investigations after one attack.

The bladder is lined with a delicate membrane of cells richly supplied with blood vessels. Cystitis is very painful because this delicate lining of the bladder becomes inflamed, and is in constant contact with acidic urine. The urethra also becomes inflamed. In a bad attack, the lining actually bleeds. Scar tissues form which heal after attacks but may open again and bleed later.

Cystitis is normally caused by bacteria getting into the bladder and multiplying. The main bacterium which causes cystitis is E. coli (Escherichia coliform) which lives in the bowel. This is the main contaminant in impure water and is often the cause of holiday diarrhoea. E. coli in a suitable environment – and human urine is at just the right temperature and contains just the right substances to encourage it – multiplies extremely rapidly.

Sex is a common cause
Sexual intercourse can be a trigger for cystitis because the thrusting actions of the penis in the vagina can force the germs or bacteria on the skin up into the urethra. The warm, moist secretions and swelling of the tissues caused by sexual arousal in the woman also help the growth of bacteria. For many women, then, the first attack comes soon after having sexual intercourse for the first time, or after having vigorous and exciting sex at the beginning of a relationship; hence the

22

popular term 'honeymoon cystitis'.

More unusual sexual techniques can be more likely to cause cystitis. The recent massive survey 'Sexual behaviour in Britain' showed that about one eighth of both men and women had tried anal sex, meaning full penetration of the penis into the anus. Of course, since anal sex is actually illegal in England and Wales, some people may not have admitted to it, and the real incidence may be higher. Anal intercourse is more common among people under forty-five, and especially those aged eighteen to twenty-four. However, many more couples, rather than having full anal intercourse, will insert a finger into the anus or stimulate the anus to cause sexual pleasure. This means that unless great care is taken, contamination with harmful bacteria from the gut is almost a certainty.

Any woman who has suffered from cystitis or wishes to avoid it should ask for her partner's cooperation in making sure that if he touches or penetrates the anus with his hand, finger or penis, he should then avoid touching the vaginal area with it. Ideally, if you have full anal sex the man should wear a condom, which he can discard afterwards. Anal intercourse followed straight away by vaginal intercourse should never be attempted as the risk of causing infections of both the vagina and the bladder is too great.

Vaginal tampons and contraceptive diaphragms can also lead to a tendency to cystitis in some women, for two reasons. First, if care is not taken in inserting them bacteria can be introduced into the vagina where they breed and are thus more likely to spread to the urethra, especially during sex. Second, the cap and tampon tend to press against the urethra and make it more difficult to empty the bladder completely. Anyone who has tried to pee in a hurry with a full bladder with a super tampon in place will know what this means – 'like pouring water from a furred-up kettle', as one woman put it. The bladder may not be completely emptied so stale urine –

perhaps infected with bacteria – is left behind to contaminate the urine.

Another reason why tampons may cause cystitis is their strings. These may move around, rubbing first against the anal region and then against the urethra. Some women change to external sanitary towels because of this, but these may also help the spread of bacteria as the warm, wet tissue is an ideal breeding ground.

Soft loo paper may also not help. Tiny damp pieces may get left behind after you've wiped yourself, get contaminated with bacteria, and move around inside your pants, taking the germs with them.

Don't hang on!

Not going to pee regularly can also cause problems. Stale urine is left in the bladder for long periods, making it easier for germs to multiply. If the bladder becomes over-full, urine collects in the ureters, and this means that if you have bacteria in the urine this can make it easier for the bacteria to spread up to the kidneys. After you have emptied the bladder, urine then runs from the ureters back into the bladder and collects there. This is why, as you may have noticed, you often need to pee again quite soon after peeing with a very full bladder.

Another cause of cystitis is not drinking enough. If you drink frequently, your kidneys will produce a lot of dilute urine and you will need to pee quite frequently. This means that any harmful bacteria are regularly flushed out of the bladder. Weak urine forms a less favourable breeding ground for bacteria than strong urine, so again, this tends to keep cystitis at bay.

In our modern, stressed lives, women often find they do not take time to go to the loo as soon as they want to, and do not take time to drink regularly. Also, the drinks we tend to take socially are coffee, tea and alcoholic drinks, all of which are liable to aggravate cystitis. Tea, coffee and alcohol all tend to dehydrate the body and irritate the bladder.

Fashion or common sense?
Modern clothing can also be a problem. Close-fitting nylon underwear and tights stop air circulating and the skin from breathing and keep the area damp and moist, providing a good breeding ground for germs. Tight, hard jeans or trousers can rub against the opening of the urethra and cause soreness and irritation, making the tissues swell and harbour bacteria and possibly damaging the skin, again making it easier for bacteria to invade. Many women notice they have less trouble from cystitis in the summer when they wear thin cotton pants and cotton skirts or dresses.

Some women suffer from cystitis which is not caused by an invading bacteria. They are thought usually to have particularly sensitive bladder and urethral linings. Some women are allergic to chemicals in soaps, bubble baths, spermicidal creams or vaginal deodorants, talcum powder, chlorine (as found in swimming pools) and certain washing powders. Certain spicy or acidic foods can trigger attacks in sensitive people. Chilli powder, citrus fruits such as oranges and grapefruit, vinegar and wine can all cause the urine to become acidic and affect the bladder lining.

The act of sex can also cause irritation to the urethra producing symptoms of cystitis with no bacteria involved.

Sometimes letting the lower part of the body become chilled, by sitting on a cold surface or sitting in a damp swimming costume, can cause an attack of cystitis (hence the old-fashioned term 'a chill on the bladder').

'Complicated' urinary tract infections and pyelonephritis
Although normally an attack of cystitis is restricted to the urethra and bladder, the infection can, in severe cases, ascend

up the ureters and into the kidneys. This occurs in a very small percentage of cases and is usually linked to another problem in the urinary system. In severe cases it can cause an infection of the kidneys – pyelonephritis. The symptoms are:

★ Chills
★ Fever
★ Pain in the side or back
★ Nausea and vomiting
★ A sense of wanting to pee urgently
★ Frequent urination

These symptoms vary from one person to another. Some people find they can continue with their day-to-day activities, while others suffer so much pain that they may be incapacitated and require admission to hospital. Pyelonephritis can become life-threatening because of the potential spread of bacteria from the kidneys into the bloodstream, so urgent diagnosis and antibiotic therapy are needed.

In about 75–85% of upper urinary tract infections the bacterium E. coli is the cause, the remainder being due to Klebsiella, Proteus sp or, more rarely, streptococci, staphylococci, or others. Once infection has spread to the kidneys it can be difficult to treat because the structure of the kidney makes it difficult for white blood cells and other immune system agents to penetrate.

An upper urinary tract infection is usually accompanied by cystitis and can be detected by blood and pus cells in the urine.

Sometimes kidney infections can develop into a perinephric abscess, usually when the bacterium Staphylococcus aureus is involved. In this condition there is marked pain and tenderness in the region of the kidneys and there may be swelling on the affected side. The sufferer often has a high fever and is often extremely ill. Unlike pyelonephritis, there are no pus cells or organisms in the urine. A perinephric abscess requires hospital admission and surgical drainage.

Another problem with pyelonephritis is that the kidneys are very delicate organs, and cystitis in children can cause kidney damage and scarring, resulting in permanent kidney problems. If there are no abnormalities in the urinary tract, pyelonephritis in adults does not normally lead to serious chronic renal disease. If there are recurrent urinary tract infections, however, it is rather a different story. The risk, albeit small, that an attack of cystitis might, if neglected, lead to kidney problems means that you must always take it very seriously especially if you know that your kidneys are already scarred.

Complicated urinary tract infections account for only about 10% of all urinary tract infections, and are most commonly found in older people. The most common cause in a man is prostate problems, and in a woman, kidney stones or an underlying abnormality of the urinary tract.

Sometimes chronic cystitis will involve the Skene's glands, tiny glands at the opening of the urethra. Sometimes you think you are cured, but during sexual intercourse the glands are squeezed and release some pus, which starts the cystitis symptoms up again. Occasionally the Skene's glands are removed in an operation, though this is controversial.

Medical causes of cystitis

Repeated cystitis can sometimes be traced back to some underlying cause, an abnormality or weakness in the urinary system, so women who have several attacks of cystitis should have a medical examination and investigations to make sure this is not the case. If abnormalities are identified they need to be dealt with appropriately.

The main problems of the urinary system which may lead to cystitis are bladder cysts, kidney stones, a faulty valve at the outlet of the kidney or at the junction of the ureter and bladder. Damage to the urethra, sometimes caused during labour, can cause a narrowing of the urethra and problems in emptying the bladder, also leading to cystitis.

Diabetes can result in sugar in the urine which encourages the growth of bacteria and may lead to cystitis.

HORMONAL CAUSES

Changes in the woman's hormones may lead to cystitis. This is why some women get cystitis in pregnancy and others after the menopause. The lower part of the urethra is closely linked to the vagina. Declining oestrogen levels after the menopause affects both the vaginal walls and the urethra, making it more liable to irritation and infection. Usually a three-month course of hormone replacement therapy will clear up the problem.

INTERSTITIAL CYSTITIS

Interstitial cystitis is the subject of considerable controversy among doctors. Some believe that it is a newly discovered disease, others are doubtful that it exists at all. Some people cynically believe that interstitial cystitis is a catch-all term used by doctors for women who have all the symptoms of cystitis, but in whom no bacterial infection can be found.

According to an American research paper by Ratner, Slade and Greene, 'interstitial cystitis is a painful and debilitating bladder disease which affects a sizable proportion of those women with symptoms of cystitis in whom no bacteria can be found.' It estimates that there are 450,000 women in the United States affected by it. Although men can also get it, 90% of sufferers are women. The condition was formerly thought to affect mainly post-menopausal women, but it is now realised that it occurs in women of all ages; 25% of women with this condition are under thirty.

Interstitial cystitis has only been recognised recently and now a great deal of research is being carried out into it, to try to find out exactly what it is and what causes it, and, therefore, how it can be prevented and treated. It is thought now that this form of cystitis may be some kind of auto-immune disease, where cells in the body's own immune system attack a vulnerable place. This is borne out by the fact that the inflamed bladder wall contains large numbers of cells called mast cells which are involved in allergic responses such as asthma.

Some doctors now think that many women in the past suffered for years, going repeatedly to their doctors with symptoms of cystitis only to be told that there were no bacteria in their urine and that it was all in their head. They were told that they had 'urethral syndrome' or 'trigonitis', an inflammation of the bladder sphincter, or that they had a 'sensitive bladder'. A doctor researching into cystitis in the 1980s had this to say about women with the 'urethral syndrome': 'Women with the urethral syndrome tend to suffer from anxiety, have relationship problems, and generally feel less healthy.' In the past, women with symptoms of cystitis whose bacterial urine count was negative received treatments such as dilatation of the urethra and steroid injections into the urethra, none of which could be shown to have much, if any, effect.

The symptoms of interstitial cystitis are similar to those of bacterial cystitis. There is pelvic pain and pressure, and a frequent need to urinate, possibly as often as sixty to eighty times a day. Women with interstitial cystitis often complain of pain during and after sexual intercourse.

One recent study of interstitial cystitis showed that 44% of the sufferers had had a hysterectomy, and 38% had strong sensitivities or allergic reactions to medication. More than 60% of the women said that they were unable to enjoy usual activities or were excessively fatigued, and 54% reported depression. Travel, employment, leisure activities and sleeping were adversely affected in 80% of sufferers.

Because this condition is not caused by bacteria, there is no simple and straightforward cure. Many of the precautions taken to prevent or cope with an attack of conventional cystitis work well (see below).

It's worth noting that a link has been made between the anti-arthritis drug tiaprofenic acid (Surgam) and interstitial cystitis.

Angela Kilmartin, the self-help expert on cystitis, is, however, cynical about the condition. She believes that interstitial cystitis is in fact an inflamed bladder caused by medical treatments such as urethral and bladder dilatation, the washing of the bladder with chemicals, and other interventions, as well as by repeated cystitis attacks. She notes that the condition is more common in the United States, where she believes far more aggressive treatment was used for recurrent cystitis than in Britain. She believes that doctors would rather 'invent' a new condition than admit to the mistakes of the past. Unfortunately, if this were true much of the medical treatment on offer for interstitial cystitis appears to be the kind of treatment which Angela Kilmartin believes may have been responsible for it in the first place.

Why do some women go on getting cystitis?

There is no doubt that some women are unlucky and are prone to constant attacks of cystitis. Angela Kilmartin says that it may be a matter of personal anatomy, but this is unlikely; while some women may have small differences in the distance between anus and urethra it's unlikely to be significant. Women with external piles may find it harder to clean the anal area thoroughly and this may lead to cystitis.

It is probable that there are immune factors at work. There is evidence that the cells lining the urethra of some women may be more 'sticky' to bacteria than that of others. The cells of their vaginal walls also appear to harbour these bugs more readily, and the bacteria travel from the anus to the urethra via the vagina. This is probably the most convincing reason why cystitis never attacks some women, even though they are highly sexually active and not scrupulous about personal hygiene, while others suffer again and again despite all their precautions.

HOW TO TREAT IT

Visiting your GP – what to expect

The usual medical cure for an attack of cystitis is a course of antibiotics. Generally a simple on-the-spot urine test can be carried out which will confirm that there is a urinary tract infection. The doctor should send the sample away to test for the specific bacterium which is causing the problem, but in the meantime will probably prescribe an antibiotic, which is hopefully the correct one to solve the problem. If the test shows later – it usually takes thirty-six hours to check on which kind of bacterium it is – that you are taking the wrong antibiotic, the doctor should contact you and give you a new prescription.

It is important to give women an antibiotic straight away. Far too many women have been made to suffer unnecessarily in the past until the result of their urine test came back.

If you have several episodes, or if you have really severe attacks of cystitis with blood in the urine, your GP will probably suggest a hospital appointment and further investigations. These may be done to make sure that you do not have some medical problem which might be the cause of your repeat attacks.

Medical investigation and diagnosis

BLOOD TESTS

The doctor may carry out a blood test. A few millilitres of blood will be withdrawn from your arm with a syringe. The blood sample is then tested in a hospital laboratory for a shortage of blood cells which might indicate anaemia (possible if you have been losing blood in the urine), and the presence of white blood cells, which indicate an infection. Tests are also carried out to see whether you may have a kidney problem.

Urine tests

You will be asked to provide a fresh mid-stream urine sample. You will usually be given a tissue to wipe the area around the urethra to make sure the sample will not be contaminated by any germs on the skin. You then start peeing, stop the flow, collect the middle part of the stream in the container you are given, and then finish peeing. The idea is that the sample will contain only urine which has been in the bladder and will not be contaminated by germs which might be hanging around at the urethral opening or on the skin.

The urine will be tested for the presence of protein, which may indicate kidney problems, and the acidity of the urine will also be measured. First the pathologist or technician will examine a drop of urine under a microscope. This will show the presence of pus, bacteria and any blood cells (there may be small amounts of blood not visible to the eye). Sometimes a biological stain is added to help show up and identify the bacteria. Tests can also be carried out to detect white blood cells in the urine, which are also a good indication that there is an infection.

To identify the exact strain of bacterium and which antibiotic it is sensitive to, the urine is plated out onto petri dishes with a special culture medium ideal for growing bacteria. After twenty-four hours, the plates are checked to see if the bacteria have grown. Antibiotics are then added, and another 12–24 hours allowed to see whether the antibiotic kills or stops the growth of bacteria. The end result, therefore, is a minimum of thirty-six hours, which is why most doctors will start you on antibiotic therapy as soon as cystitis is diagnosed, rather than waiting for the result.

Bacteria are divided into two main groups – 'Gram negative' and 'Gram positive'. The Gram stain is a reliable, simple test to identify these strains, which respond to different antibiotics. E. coli and Proteus are both Gram negative; occasionally cystitis can be caused by a Gram positive bacterium such as Staphylococcus aureus.

Routinely, a bacterial count of 10^5 (100,000 per ml) is considered significant, but in children or old people a count of 10^4 may be considered worth treating. However, Dr James Malone Lee at St Pancras hospital says that in fact there is only about a 50% chance of getting a significant bacterial count from urine even when an infection is present. Often bacteria do not survive the long wait and journey from the GP's surgery to the laboratory.

Further, if a woman has been drinking a great deal to alleviate symptoms her urine may be too dilute to show a significant count. Dr Lee also believes that looking for a count of 10^5 per ml is arbitrary and far too high. He feels this is an acceptable level if there are no symptoms, but if the woman has symptoms, and especially severe ones, then a count of 10^4 or even 10^2 should be considered positive. Unfortunately most laboratory tests are not sensitive enough to detect this. It may be worth taking a mid-stream sample from the very first urine of the day because this will be the most concentrated and gives the greatest opportunity to find enough bacteria.

LOOKING AT THE BLADDER

This is a minor operation known as a '**cystoscopy**' in which a doctor passes a viewing instrument through the urethra into the bladder to look at the bladder lining. You may be given a general anaesthetic or a sedative and local anaesthetic contained in a jelly. Your legs are placed in stirrups and a catheter inserted to drain the bladder of urine. The cystoscope is then inserted and sterile solution is passed into the bladder via the tube. The surgeon is able to view the bladder walls with a lens via a fibre optic cable.

The surgeon can check the urethra and bladder for inflammation, small growths like cysts, bladder stones or any irregularities of the bladder wall which might harbour micro-organisms which cause cystitis. Biopsies can also be taken.

It is also possible to view the ureters directly in a continuation of this procedure, if the problem is thought to be in the kidneys. Urine samples can be taken from each tube.

LOOKING AT THE KIDNEYS

A test known as an **intravenous pyelogram** (**IVP**) can be carried out in cases of recurrent cystitis. The test is carried out in an X-Ray department, and works by injecting a 'contrast medium' into your arm and waiting for the kidneys to concentrate and excrete it. This can then be viewed by a series of X-Rays which show the kidneys and urinary system at work.

You are usually told not to drink anything for a few hours before the test is done so that only a little urine is passing through the kidneys.

The contrast medium, which contains radioactive iodine and is opaque to X-Rays, is a liquid which is injected slowly into a vein in your arm. This should not be painful, but most people say that it is quite unpleasant. Many people say they either have a 'pins and needles' sensation in the muscles of the upper and lower arm and sometimes the lower leg as the dye is injected, or they experience a warm flush all over. Some people say that they feel quite ill for a while after the test is done.

Harriet had the test done when a faulty kidney valve was suspected. 'The worst aspect of it was having to lie still for about three hours while the test was done,' she recalls. 'I did have a hot feeling when the dye was injected but it didn't really hurt. The nurses did warn me about that and they were very nice and supportive.

'They didn't volunteer much information; I had to ask them if it was all right for me to breast-feed afterwards, and then they realised that I shouldn't feed the baby for twenty-four hours. They didn't warn me about any risks or side-effects or that it was rather a mistake for me to have decided to walk home afterwards. In fact I couldn't get home and had to ask a woman on the street to help me because I felt terribly dizzy.'

Most people sail through the investigation with no problem. Occasionally people can have an allergic reaction to the dye, and this can be serious. Very rarely, people have died following the test. However, if you do have a kidney problem, the chances are that if it is untreated kidney damage may result and in the worst case scenario it could mean kidney failure, dialysis and a kidney transplant. You should discuss the risks and benefits of having this investigation with your specialist.

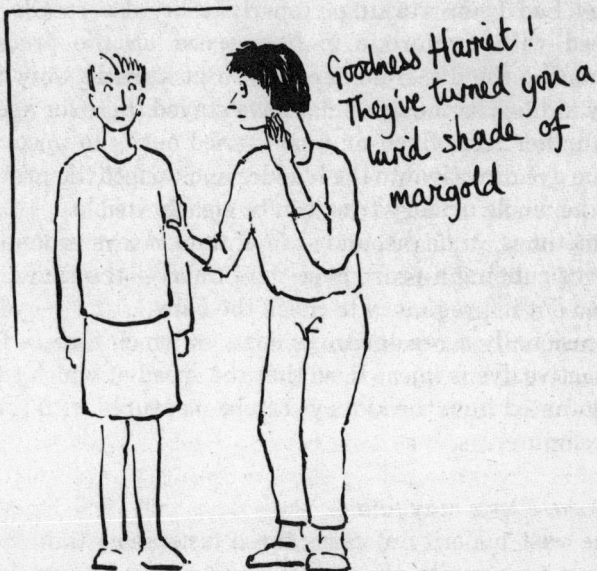

Goodness Harriet! They've turned you a lurid shade of marigold

As the dye is concentrated by the kidneys a shadow will show up on the X-Ray outlining the shape of the kidneys. As the dye passes out of the kidneys, then down the ureters into the bladder, the speed with which this happens will be made clear, and it will be obvious if there is any difference in the functioning of the two kidneys. The opaque dye will be visible in the bladder, and here it will be obvious whether there are any deformations of the wall of the bladder, and whether the valves at the entrance to the bladder work properly, preventing urine from leaking back into the ureters, 'reflux' in medical jargon. Finally, the effectiveness of the bladder can be seen when the woman urinates, and whether there is any stale urine left behind in the bladder afterwards.

Harriet experienced a pain in her back, 'around the kidneys, as if it hurt when the radioactive dye was being forced through. I don't know whether it would have hurt if my kidney had been working properly.' She also recalls being injected with a diuretic to help speed up the process of eliminating the dye from her body. 'But it didn't work in the faulty kidney, so the dye must have stayed there for ages.'

A further test which may be carried out is to inject radio opaque dye directly into the bladder and up into the ureters so that the whole urinary tract can be clearly visible.

Sometimes an ultrasound scan of the kidneys is done. This involves rubbing a probe over the tummy – the same test is carried out in pregnancy to check the baby.

Occasionally a **renogram** is done, in which a more highly radioactive dye is injected, so that the speed at which the dye is eliminated from the kidneys can be measured with the help of a computer.

What these tests may find
In the vast majority of cases these tests show that there is nothing wrong with the kidneys or urinary system. In this case, the woman can be reassured that the normal methods of

treating cystitis should be sufficient.

In some cases, however, congenital or mechanical abnormalities are found. Among these are faulty valves where the ureters enter the bladder, allowing urine to reflux back from the bladder into the ureters. This is usually treated by surgery to correct the faulty valve.

Another problem is a swelling of the bladder wall, known as a diverticulum, which allows stagnant urine to pool in it. This can be congenital, or is sometimes caused when the bladder has been overstretched, usually when there has been an obstruction to its outflow. This is more common in men who suffer an enlarged prostate gland than in women. In women, the urethra can sometimes be traumatised during childbirth and there may be a stricture, or narrowing of the urethra, which prevents the easy flow of urine to the outside. The woman may experience difficulty in peeing, and may not empty her bladder completely, thus allowing urine to remain behind encouraging infection. This can usually be cured by a simple operation to stretch the urethra. The operation is normally done as a day-care operation under local anaesthetic.

Another problem affecting the bladder is after there has been a prolapse of the womb. This may cause pressure on the bladder, or there may be a prolapse of the bladder itself. A prolapse is caused when the pelvic muscles keeping the organs in place are weakened, and the organs tend to sag, bulging down into the vaginal canal.

If the bladder prolapses, there may be a kink in the urethra, which impedes the flow of urine. A prolapse of the bladder, where it sags into the vaginal canal, is called a cystocele. A lump or bulge just inside the vaginal opening may be felt. A woman with a large cystocele will have difficulty emptying her bladder properly. As part of the bladder will sag down below the upper end of the urethra, urine cannot drain from the area and remains behind. This gives the woman the sensation of still wanting to pee after she has finished urinating. Often the symptoms are worse at bedtime; she empties her bladder, lies down, and immediately feels she wants to go again. Because of the stagnant urine left behind in the bladder, women with cystoceles are much more likely to suffer from recurrent attacks of cystitis.

A prolapsed womb can also cause the same problem, as the sagging womb tends to press on the bladder, pushing it out of shape and also making it hard for the woman to empty her bladder.

Prolapses are usually caused by trauma done to the tissues during childbirth. They are becoming less common today, for several reasons. First, better obstetric care and the availability of Caesarian sections in complicated deliveries mean that fewer women experience a long and difficult second stage in labour, straining and pushing for hours to deliver the baby. Secondly, the increase in popularity of breast-feeding in recent years means that the womb contracts down much more quickly after the delivery of a baby and the pubococcus muscle, which acts as a sling across the lower pelvis holding the female organs in their place, is strengthened by involuntary contractions when the baby sucks at the breast.

Exercising the pubococcus muscle yourself – doing your 'pelvic floor exercises' – is also a good way of preventing prolapses occurring; more of this on page 138.

If a prolapse is the problem, an operation can usually be carried out to correct it, with varying degrees of success. The organs are put back into their original places and repairs of the muscles can keep them there. Usually the operation requires a few days' stay in hospital.

Occasionally a cystoscopy will reveal a rare form of cystitis, known as Hunner's cystitis or interstitial cystitis. This condition has only been recognised fairly recently and is found when symptoms of cystitis are present but when no bacteria seem to be present in the urine. On examination with a cystoscope, the bladder lining will be seen to be inflamed.

Kidney stones are another cause of obstruction in the urinary system, and sometimes lead to cystitis. The stones can move down the ureters, causing very severe pain. They can usually be removed by surgery.

Bladder stones can cause similar problems. Stagnant urine can become a source of an infection. The infection makes the urine more alkaline, and this may encourage calcium salts in the urine to crystallise round an impurity, resulting in a bladder stone which, if not expelled, will increase in size until it causes symptoms. Today bladder stones can be destroyed by a process called a lithotripsy, where an instrument is passed through the urethra into the bladder and then grinds them. Occasionally they can get very big, the size of an orange, and need to be removed by open surgery.

What if an infection is not found?

In a certain proportion of women who go to their doctor with symptoms of cystitis, no bacteria will be found. Of course, this may be because the bacterial culture didn't grow enough bacteria to be considered an infection (see page 33). It's a good idea to repeat the tests. If all your urine tests prove negative, however, inflammation of the urethra may be caused by irritants such as perfumed soaps and deodorants, highly perfumed washing powders or talcum powders, which irritate the entrance to the urethra and cause symptoms of urgency and a frequent need to pee. Sometimes these symptoms can also be caused by sexual intercourse or by a thrush infection (see Chapter 2).

Some women suffer from an irritability of the bladder, in which the complicated signals which go from the stretched bladder wall to the brain, saying that you need to pee, respond too readily when the bladder is not full. Women who suffer from this problem can be treated by drugs, or can be taught, to some extent, to 'retrain' the bladder.

After having a baby, some women have got into the habit of peeing very frequently, because the baby's head pressing on the bladder means the bladder can hold less. After giving birth, the bladder still signals that it is full when it is carrying less volume, and so the woman gets into the habit of peeing frequently, which can become a great nuisance for her. Retraining yourself to go for longer intervals between peeing can help your bladder get back to normal. Some women, afraid of cystitis, constantly drink too many fluids and in consequence overwork the bladder and cause it to become irritable.

The beginning of a period can also cause bladder irritability, frequent peeing as the body expels the excess fluids some women accumulate before menstruation, and back pain, which can all seem like the beginning of a cystitis attack, and some women can mistake blood from the vagina for blood in urine. However, very few women who have had a severe attack of cystitis will confuse anything else with it.

Another possibility is what is now termed 'interstitial cystitis' (see page 28).

TREATMENT

Antibiotics
If it's your first attack of cystitis, you will probably be given a short course of antibiotics. If it's recurrent, you will usually be prescribed a full five- to ten-day course of antibiotics at a standard dose. The most common bacterium in cystitis is E. coli, which is responsible for an estimated 80–90% of uncomplicated urinary tract infections. Following this is the bacterium Staphylococcus saprophyticus, which accounts for most of the remaining infections. Proteus is another bacterium which is sometimes the cause; it is often linked to kidney stones. Proteus often has a strong, distinctive smell which can

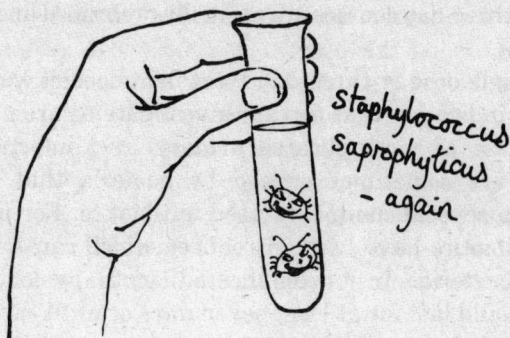

Staphylococcus
saprophyticus
– again

be detected in the urine; women say that it smells like rotten fish.

The usual antibiotics prescribed are those which are effective against these bacteria. These include **trimethoprim** (brand names **Ipral**, **Monotrim**, **Trimopan**), **co-trimoxazole** (**Septrin**, **Chemotrim**), **ampicillin** (**Penbritin**), **amoxycillin** (**Amoxyl**).

Nitrofurantoin (**Furadantin**, **Macrodantin**, **Urantoin**) is familiar to many cystitis sufferers, as it has a good record in clearing up 'honeymoon' cystitis and is also sometimes used for long-term, low-dose treatment. For patients with penicillin sensitivity, **nalidixic acid** (**Mictral**, **Negram**, **Uribin**) can be very useful. Many strains of E. coli are sensitive to **sulphonamides** (for example, **Gantrisin**, **Kelfizine**, and **Urolucosil**), so these are sometimes prescribed.

It is now believed by many doctors that the traditional five-day course of antibiotics for cystitis is extravagant. There is no convincing evidence that a long course of medication is more effective than a short one, and in fact, the use of a single dose therapy is gaining support. The single dose treatment usually prescribed by doctors consists of 600mg of trimethoprim, 1.92g co-trimoxazole, 3g fosfomycin trometamol and the 4-quinolones. Otherwise three-day courses are normally prescribed and should be sufficient.

If the single dose or three-day treatment doesn't work, this may be an indication that further investigations are needed.

In the case of a complicated urinary tract infection, the infections are sometimes caused by bacteria that can be resistant to several commonly used antibiotics. Fortunately, newer antibiotics have been introduced which can kill these resistant bacteria. In uncomplicated acute pyelonephritis therapy should last for at least seven days or until three days after the fever has gone. If there is some other complication, a longer course of antibiotic therapy may be required to ensure that the infection won't return, usually for at least 10–14 days until the fever has subsided or any complication identified, such as a kidney stone, has been dealt with.

For serious infections, or people in hospital, antibiotics can be given by injection or through an intravenous drip. Doctors watch patients with complicated urinary tract infections very closely, and ask them to return for frequent follow-up visits.

SIDE-EFFECTS

All drugs have side-effects and while antibiotics are usually fairly safe, it's worth knowing that there can be adverse reactions to them.

Many antibiotics have minor side-effects such as nausea or mild diarrhoea, but in some cases there are more serious reactions. Penicillin hypersensitivity is well known. It usually first manifests itself as a rash, sometimes a raised, itchy rash, and sometimes a flat, bright red one. If this happens you should immediately inform your doctor, who will advise you to stop taking the penicillin. Once you have had an adverse reaction you should not take penicillin again, as there are alternative effective antibiotics available. Once you are sensitised to penicillin, the next reaction may be more severe and can even be fatal, which is why doctors always ask before prescribing whether you are sensitive to penicillin.

Co-trimoxazole (**Septrin**, **Chemotrim**) consists of two drugs, sulphamethoxazole (a sulphonamide) and trimethoprim. Adverse reactions to either one of these drugs can occur. Nausea, vomiting, diarrhoea, headache, dizziness, drug fever and skin rashes are all uncommon, but do happen. Very rarely they may produce a severe disorder of the skin and mucous membranes which may be fatal in 25% of cases.

Septrin in particular has received some publicity recently because of these rare and fatal side-effects. Septrin was very heavily advertised and promoted in the medical press for cystitis, and some people are concerned that this publicity led doctors to prescribe Septrin first over other drugs which are available. Do discuss the antibiotic you take with your doctor and ask about risks and side-effects. It's your body and you have a right to know.

If you are pregnant, or might be pregnant, point this out to your doctor. **Co-trimoxazole** should never be prescribed to pregnant women. It should also be given with caution to breast-feeding mothers.

TAKING THE ANTIBIOTICS

More women nowadays are being prescribed a single dose of antibiotic, which avoids the problem of remembering to take the tablets. If you are taking a longer course, it is very important that you take the antibiotics regularly and as evenly spaced as possible throughout the day. If you are one of those people who is always forgetting to take pills, get somebody to remind you, or set a clock, watch or calculator alarm to go off regularly to remind you. If you forget whether you've taken one or not, count the pills so that you know where you are.

Always remember to finish the course. The antibiotics may work quickly and the symptoms be alleviated in a day or two, but it's important to go on taking the pills. If you stop too soon, some bacteria will remain and may multiply again, and the infection will flare up again. What is more, the bacteria which remain may be those which are more resistant to the drug, so you may get a flare-up of resistant bacteria, which will be much harder to treat.

Women with recurrent cystitis may be put on a low dose of antibiotic for three months or more to prevent a recurrence. The most effective drugs for this type of treatment include nitro-furantoin 50mg, trimethoprim 100mg and norfloxacin 200mg, given at night. More recent studies show that a dose taken on alternate nights or three times a week is just as effective. Other doctors suggest that you keep a small supply of antibiotics so that you can take a tablet at the first symptoms and with any luck prevent an infection. Some doctors suggest that if the cystitis always occurs after you have sex, you should take a tablet then; but not to be advised if you have frequent sex! Ask your doctor what the ideal dosage is.

After several episodes of acute cystitis, which played havoc with Nora's work and with her love life, she always carried around a bottle of antibiotics. As soon as the cystitis started, she would take a tablet. 'I tried everything else, all the natural remedies, drinking pints of water, but nothing else worked. Taking antibiotics on and off all the time was the only way I could keep it at bay and stay sane.'

Other treatments
In interstitial cystitis, antibiotic therapy will have no effect. There are some treatments for this as yet little understood disease which have been suggested for some sufferers:

★ **Bladder distension**, in which the bladder is distended while under regional or general anaesthetic.
★ Washing the bladder with a number of therapeutic drugs, such as **Dimethyl sulfoxide**, and **oxychlorosene sodium**,

which are believed to reduce inflammation.

★ Medications: women are often prescribed a variety of non-steroidal anti-inflammatory medications, anti-spasmodics and anti-histamines. **Sodium pentosan-polyphosphate** is believed to coat the bladder wall and protect it from irritants in the urine. In a trial, 32% of people taking the drug showed an improvement in symptoms, compared with 16% who took a placebo. **Nalmefene** is another drug which is currently undergoing trials.

★ **Anti-depressants** are also often prescribed, together with a variety of painkillers.

★ Elimination of spicy foods, alcohol, citrus fruits and tomatoes seem to alleviate symptoms in many cases (see below for hints on diet).

There are some who believe that these treatments may actually do more harm than good, by further irritating and interfering with the bladder.

Relieving the symptoms
One of the most important things you can do when you get an attack of cystitis is to **drink**. Drinking plenty of water will help dilute the urine in the bladder, making it less acid and less painful when you pee. It will also mean you keep emptying your bladder, flushing the harmful bacteria out of your body.

As any cystitis sufferer knows, the very worst thing is sitting on the loo feeling as if you're dying to pee when there is nothing there to pee out, and every little dribble feels like razor-sharp glass. However, some doctors think that women who literally drink pints and pints of fluid continually with an attack may simply be causing the bladder to overwork and diluting the antibiotics, thus making them less effective. Dr James Malone Lee at St Pancras hospital points out that 80% of cases of cystitis will get better by themselves, so women sometimes think they have cured the infection when it would have been defeated by the body's defences anyway. He also points out that bacteria can invade the cells of the bladder wall and therefore cannot be washed away by drinking fluids. Do drink to relieve symptoms, certainly, but don't try to wash yourself away completely!

You can also help by making the urine more acid or more alkaline in order to help kill off the bacteria. Most bacteria have a preferred degree of acidity or alkalinity in which they best survive. The measure of the acid/alkali balance is known as pH, with low pH being acid and high pH alkaline. The pH range of normal urine is between about pH 4.6 to 7.25, and the most common bacteria which causes cystitis, E. coli, prefers a pH of between 6 and 7.

One natural remedy is **cranberry juice**. This is highly acid and helps kill bacteria as well as alleviating the symptoms. Pure cranberry juice on its own without sugar is best if you can get it. If you are prone to cystitis always keep it in the house.

Many women prefer to use an alkaline remedy, as the alkali also tends to neutralise the acid made by the bacteria and to alleviate the stinging when you pee. Pain on passing urine can also be relieved by taking **sodium bicarbonate** (5–10g daily in divided doses) or **sodium or potassium citrate** (3–6g every six hours). The latter was prescribed as the mist. pot. cit. in hospitals, and many cystitis sufferers will remember it only too well. It was sometimes given with hyoscine (hyocyamus), to prevent nausea. You are meant to measure out 10ml of this greenish fluid and drink it in water three times a day; it tastes absolutely disgusting. Though it's now fifteen years since I had my last cystitis attack, I can still remember its vile taste to this day.

Various over-the-counter remedies of this sort are available, such as **Cystemme**, which contains sodium citrate and sodium bicarbonate. When dissolved in water the sachet contents form a fizzy lemon-flavoured drink. Each sachet contains about 4g of sodium citrate, and should be used with caution in pregnancy.

Claire developed an attack of cystitis very suddenly one evening, and, reluctant to call the doctor, sent her husband out to buy one of the proprietary brands of cystitis-relieving sachets. 'It was screamingly painful, awful, I was peeing dark red blood and it was agony. Within two hours of taking the sachet I felt much, much better. I went to see my doctor in the morning and he prescribed antibiotics to make sure there weren't any lingering bacteria left, but I'm convinced the highly alkaline urine did the trick and killed off most of the infection.'

If you don't have any of these alkaline drinks available, pure water is best. **Barley water** can be helpful; you can make your own by simmering a handful of organic whole barley in a pint of water for an hour with a whole lemon cut into pieces. Some **herb infusions** are helpful; parsley is one. Beware of drinking too much tea or coffee, as these can irritate the already inflamed and irritated bladder.

You can also keep your diet alkaline, by eating fruit, vegetables and whole grains, and by avoiding all acid foods and drinks such as citrus foods. Also avoid alcohol, which is dehydrating and tends to concentrate the urine, making it even more painful to pee.

Acid foods to avoid:
Orange juice
Other citrus fruits and juices
Coffee
Tea
Cola drinks
Alcohol
Pepper
Spices

Apart from drinking, it's important to rest. Go to bed, and stay there. Use a hot water bottle over the bladder area and perhaps around the small of the back to ease the discomfort; raising the body's temperature in these areas will also help the body's fight against the bacteria, which like to be at body heat and not more. Keeping warm is very helpful. If you are really having trouble peeing, and it's terribly painful, run a hot bath, get in, and pee into the bath. This will be easier and feel less painful; just pee whenever you feel like it. Have a bottle of fluid by the bath and keep drinking it, and keep topping up the bath with hot water so that you don't get cold.

In a severe attack, your doctor may prescribe **Urispas** (**flavoxate hydrochloride**), taken in tablet form two or three times a day. This is an anti-spasmodic, which works on the muscle fibres throughout the urinary system, relaxing and soothing them. It is also sometimes prescribed in hospital if you are having urinary investigations such as cystoscopy.

You may also like to take your usual painkillers – aspirin, codeine, paracetamol, ibuprofen – while the attack is at its worst. Take them as instructed on the packet and don't be tempted to overdose.

HOW TO PREVENT IT

Once you've had one bad attack of cystitis, you will probably want to do everything in your power to prevent it happening again!

Safer sex
How can you avoid cystitis? 'Avoid sex,' said one sufferer wryly. Obviously this is not on the cards for most people! However, you can take certain precautions to make your sex life equally or more satisfactory without running the risk of cystitis.

Cystitis tends to flare up at the beginning of a sexual relationship. If you are in a steady relationship where both partners care for and trust one another, then you can explain the problem and ways to avoid it. In a new relationship you may have been out on a date, got hot and sweaty, and you may not have the opportunity to wash when you get back to your place or his and he is overwhelmed by passion! Talking about sex – what you like and what you don't like – may be difficult at the start of a relationship too. After all, as you fall into bed, it sounds rather feeble to say, 'I am prone to cystitis. Please can you take care not to spread any germs from my back passage around the vagina.' No, it simply doesn't work!

Many people wash after sex, but it is so much better to wash before it. A quick shower or bath before you jump into bed can greatly reduce the chance of developing cystitis. Again, this is far easier to achieve in a stable relationship than when you are starting out. Still, you can always suggest it to a new partner, without saying why. You can even make a shared bath or shower part of your foreplay, and very exciting it can be, too.

The very worst kind of sex for cystitis is when you don't enjoy it. If you don't make enough lubrication, the penis will rub against the entrance to the urethra and make it sore. If the man is not highly excited and aroused before his penis enters you, it will take him longer to reach orgasm, and this may mean an awful lot of pelvic thrusting before he reaches his climax, helping push any harmful bacteria up into the urethra and bladder. If you are at all tense, this will tend to make the whole scenario worse.

The man on top position, with his weight grinding on your pubic area, is probably the very worst for causing an attack of cystitis. Experiment with different positions which don't cause so much pressure on the vulval area. Remember, you are meant to be enjoying yourselves, and you will feel much better if you are both relaxed and spend a lot of time in gentle foreplay, relaxing and arousing one another before you start on intercourse itself. You will be better lubricated and will probably find if you do this that the time spent in penetrative sex will be much shorter, and cause much less stress to the delicate tissues.

Avoid certain kinds of sexual activity which are likely to spread germs from the area around the anus into the vagina, vulva and close to the urethral opening. These involve anal sex followed by vaginal sex, and stimulating or inserting fingers into the anus before they are used to caress the clitoris or vulval area.

However, you don't have to take part in such sexual variations to spread bacteria from the anal region into the vagina. Many men do not aim well at the vagina and rub the end of their penis around the anus before inserting it. Susie, who suffered three attacks of cystitis, found that things were much better when she took the initiative, caressing her husband's penis first and then guiding it into the vagina herself. She and her husband found they both enjoyed the woman on top position, which gave Susie more control, and found that their sex life, rather than becoming 'safer' and more boring, became more enjoyable.

One tip which has prevented many an attack of cystitis is to pee immediately after having sex. This doesn't mean you have to leap out of bed the instant you've reached orgasm – you can lie there for a while and enjoy that quiet time with your partner. But don't just lie there and go to sleep for hours. Get up and pee to flush any bacteria that may have been pushed up into the urethra out of the way before they can ascend into the bladder. It's very simple, and it really works for many women. Drinking a glass of water before making love can help.

Better personal hygiene
By now you will be aware that the main cause of cystitis is bacteria from the bowel invading the bladder. So every

woman prone to cystitis – and also those who've never had it – should take particular care with personal hygiene.

When I was a child my mother always told me that after passing a stool I should always wipe my bottom from front to back. She never explained why, but it was just one of those things I accepted without a question. I was lucky; not everyone is told this, and even if they are, it is very difficult to change a lifetime's habit. However, this simple piece of information can make all the difference to cystitis sufferers. Take care to wipe backwards, and to make sure that the area around the anus is as clean as possible. If it is difficult to clean for any reason, you can try dampening the toilet tissue and washing the area.

Angela Kilmartin, founder of the self help for cystitis movement, suggests that you should wash your anal area thoroughly after passing a stool. She suggests that after passing a stool and wiping your bottom (backwards) in the usual way, you should use soap to wash the anal area. You should then wash your hands and then fill a bottle with water and pour it gently over the front of your bottom, allowing it to trickle back over the anus and down into the toilet. You should then dab (not rub) the area dry with toilet tissue.

The idea behind the bottle washing technique is that the water travels downwards, washing the perineum in front, and drips off you at the lowest point into the loo. This means that you clean the area without allowing the possibility of bacteria being washed from the anus forward towards the vaginal and urethral openings. In many Muslim countries, women squat over a primitive lavatory and use water from a small jug to wash the region using exactly this technique. In many Asian countries, too, you use your left hand to wipe your bottom and your right hand to eat food, to reduce the possibility of contamination with faeces.

Of course, you can do this easily enough in the privacy of your own bathroom, and can keep a bottle of water in the loo for this purpose. You can also buy one of the plastic jugs Muslim women use if you live in certain areas of London where there are large ethnic minorities. However, this kind of procedure is almost impossible to follow if you are in a public lavatory. You then need to take as much care as possible to clean yourself as well as you can, and go through the whole technique when you are in a suitable environment.

If you are prone to cystitis, showers are much better than using baths, because when you shower the water runs off you in such a way that water containing E. coli from the area around the anus cannot reach the vagina or vulva. In baths there is enough water to dilute the E. coli, but take care when using a bidet, as E. coli can float around in the water and contaminate the vaginal area. Angela Kilmartin says that bidets should never be used by anyone who is prone to cystitis!

You need to incorporate simple washing routines into your life, so that they become a habit. However, don't become absolutely obsessive about hygiene, or feel guilty or dirty if, despite your precautions, you still get an attack of cystitis. Remember that it is also a good idea for the man to wash before sex, too.

Swimming
Swimming pools can be dangerous for cystitis sufferers because the chlorine in the water can kill off protective bacteria on the skin, making colonisation by harmful germs like E. coli more likely. The chlorine and other chemicals can also irritate the urethra, leading to cystitis-like symptoms. Thirdly, if you wear a damp swimming costume this will chill the area and may make it more prone to infection. One woman who had suffered from cystitis for years went swimming regularly three or four times a week. As soon as she chose a different form of exercise out of the water, her cystitis attacks ceased.

After you get out of the swimming pool, go and have a warm

shower, making sure you rinse your bottom thoroughly. Also rinse out your costume if you're going to put it back on, but, preferably, having a second costume with you for sunbathing. Sitting around in a cold, damp, chlorinated swimming costume is not good news for cystitis sufferers.

Drinking
Drink more every day!

It has been said that everyone should drink six pints of fluid every day to replace body water. However, many people today don't drink this amount. In addition, the fluids that we tend to drink are tea and coffee which are diuretic and make the body pee out more fluid. They also often have the effect of irritating the bladder. We also tend to drink alcoholic drinks, which are again diuretic and which can also make the urine acid. Soft fizzy drinks also tend to be acidic and are very sugary.

These are the very worst drinks for cystitis sufferers to take. You would be much better off drinking pure mineral water and herb teas. However, while you may not mind doing this while suffering from an attack of cystitis or recovering from one, giving up your favourite drinks is too boring. So you can:

★ Drink your tea weak. Drink fine china teas which taste delicious and can be drunk very weak rather than cheap, floor-sweeping teabags which make a strong, bitter cup.
★ Restrict coffee to the morning when the body is detoxifying itself. Drink a glass of water or fruit juice with your coffee or breakfast as well. Don't drink more than two cups of strong coffee a day.
★ Drink long alcoholic drinks such as beer, gin and tonic, etc., rather than wine or shorts. If you are drinking wine with a meal, order mineral water and drink that as well. This will quench your thirst and naturally cut down on the amount of wine you are drinking, as well as diluting it.

★ If you are at a party, drink a glass of wine or whatever is on offer at the beginning. When nobody is looking, dilute your glass with some water (this is easier with white wine). Or put in ice to make white wine cool. Finally go over to water altogether; by the end of the evening the chances are nobody will notice. Don't tell people you're not drinking; they'll make a fuss, call you a killjoy and say, 'Oh, one more glass won't do any harm.' Just say yes, and then lose the wineglass after a few sips and drink something else instead.

★ Get into the habit of drinking regularly. If you drink a lot, you will be flushing out the bladder regularly and giving less time for germs to grow. The urine will also be more dilute, making a less welcome environment for invading germs.

★ If you are drinking more, you will need to go and pee more often. Don't neglect this. Busy people like mothers at home with young children, or those in busy, stressful jobs, often neglect going to pee when they need to. The longer stale urine stays in the bladder, the easier it is for bacteria to multiply. So pop out of your meeting, or leave the children for an instant while you run up the stairs, or take a break from the word processor and go and pee!

Changing contraceptive

THE CONTRACEPTIVE CAP

Marjorie used a contraceptive cap for some years before she realised that using it was the cause of her repeated attacks of cystitis.

Anything which is inserted into the vagina can inadvertently be a source of contamination. If the cap brushes against the anal region before you insert it, you may transfer bacteria into the vagina and then, during sex, this can be transferred to your urethra. Contraceptive foams, pessaries and jellies can also be a source of contamination in the same way, so take extra care when using them.

Even if you take every care while inserting a contraceptive cap, it can still cause problems. When you put the cap in, the front rim fits under the pubic bone. Here it can press against the urethra, narrowing it and making it difficult for the woman to empty her bladder. After sex, you are meant to leave the cap in place for at least six hours. If you are having a lot of sex, then, your cap can be in place for a good proportion of every day, pressing against the urethra and causing stale urine to be left behind in the bladder.

If you think this might be happening to you, you can test it by peeing with your cap in place. Pee until you feel you've finished, and then remove the cap. Try peeing again. You may be surprised to find that there is still quite a lot of urine there.

Some women find that the same thing happens with a tampon in place. Again, someone plagued by cystitis may even be willing to swap from using tampons to using external sanitary towels. Older women may be amazed to find how much slimmer and more absorbent the modern towels are, and that they usually have adhesive to enable them to fit snugly in your pants without the need for pins, loops and belts.

THE PILL AND CYSTITIS

Contrary to a common myth, there is no evidence to suggest that the Pill increases your chance of having cystitis, and this is particularly true of the modern, low-dose Pills. Many women go on the Pill because they are becoming sexually active, because of a new relationship or because they are having sex more often and more regularly. Instead of recognising that the change in their sexual behaviour has led to cystitis, they often – erroneously – blame the Pill.

Sexual aids

Any sexual aids which you insert into the vagina could be a cause of infection. Using a vibrator may be fun, but it may also be the cause of your cystitis attacks. Stop using it for a while and see if this solves the problem. Never, ever try to insert anything into your urethra for sexual pleasure. A few women say they find this sensation irresistible, but many pay for it with an attack of cystitis!

Bath scents, bubble baths and vaginal deodorants
If you suffer from cystitis, you should avoid all these things like the plague.

Women who suffer from cystitis may use vaginal deodorants in an attempt to keep themselves clean. However, the deodorants often contain substances which irritate the skin, and swollen, irritated skin helps harbour harmful bacteria. The deodorants also tend to kill off the beneficial bacteria which live on the skin and thus allow harmful bacteria from the anal area to colonise the skin, which in turn triggers an attack of cystitis or thrush.

Highly perfumed bubble baths and bath oils also tend to have the same effect of irritating the skin, and soaking in a hot, perfumed bath may provide exactly the right environment for bacteria to get a hold. Talcum powder can cause irritation as the tiny granules can get into the urethra and cause inflammation and they are usually highly perfumed, too.

Avoid using soap on the vulval area, especially perfumed soap. Again, soap kills off the good bacteria. You can use unperfumed soap to clean round the anus. Don't leave the soap to dissolve in the bath, and take care if you use perfumed shampoo and rinse this off in the bathwater. Simple salt water (one teaspoon to one pint of water) is ideal for washing the genitals and anus.

Highly perfumed, biological washing powders can also set up skin irritation. Wash your underwear in one of the unscented, non-biological brands of powder which are sold for people with sensitive skins.

CHAPTER 2
Thrush

HOW YOU GET IT

The fungus, Candida albicans, which causes thrush lives on most people's skin. In a healthy person the fungus is kept under control by a series of checks and balances. The condition of full-blown thrush is caused by what is known as an opportunistic infection – when the organism takes advantage of any weakness in the body to take a hold. You can get thrush in the mouth, throat, gut (bowel) and in the vagina.

Thrush is a common infection when the body's immune system is run down or defences are low. It is very frequent in patients with AIDS – the Acquired Immune Deficiency Syndrome, where it frequently manifests itself in the mouth and gut. It is also sometimes a problem for people who have had drugs or treatments which lower the efficiency of the immune system – following a transplant, for example, where drugs are given to suppress the body's immune reaction which tends to try to get rid of the foreign tissue. It can be found in young babies, whose immune system is not fully developed – in the mouth and nappy area – and is also common among pregnant women, whose immune system is also less effective. It is also a modern disease linked to stress.

It is also true, however, that except in the case of infants and people who are suffering from a problem with their immune system, thrush is mainly a problem which affects women in the fertile age range. Thrush is most commonly seen in women who are aged between thirteen or fourteen and the menopause. The main part of the female body which thrush infects is the vagina. Normally the vagina and cervix – neck of the womb – produce secretions which are slightly acidic and which tend to destroy harmful bacteria, fungus and other organisms. These secretions are produced most copiously at the time of ovulation – when the ovary releases the egg – and are thought to provide a suitable environment in which the man's sperm can swim up into the womb. The secretions also act to cleanse the vaginal walls and flush out harmful organisms from the body.

After ovulation, however, the secretions tend to dry up and the vagina before a period tends to be much drier and more vulnerable. Then the menstrual blood is released, which makes the vagina more alkaline and a better breeding ground for thrush.

Recently a lot of attention has been focused on the possibility that an overgrowth of thrush in the gut can be responsible for a number of symptoms such as bloatedness, indigestion, chronic fatigue and general poor health. Certainly the fungus is usually present in the gut, together with other harmless bacteria, but it is normally kept in check.

Both the gut and the vagina should be inhabited by 'friendly' bacteria, the lactobacilli, which tend to convert sugar to lactic acid, creating an environment which is hostile to thrush. If these bacteria are killed off or replaced by other, more harmful bacteria, thrush can grow unchecked.

One of the main causes of thrush is frequent use of antibiotics, and especially the broad-spectrum antibiotics which kill a wide range of bacteria. As well as killing the harmful bacteria which are causing the disease being treated, the antibiotics kill off the normal bacteria which live on the skin, in the vagina and in the digestive tract. Once they are knocked out by antibiotics, there is nothing to stop the thrush from reproducing and running rampant. Long courses of broad-spectrum antibiotics to treat acne can be a nightmare for those who are prone to thrush.

Hormonal changes can also trigger an attack of thrush. Recent research has shown that the organism which causes thrush can attach itself to molecules of oestrogen and progesterone, so high levels of these hormones may be the cause of the problem. Another theory is that an increase in the level of oestrogen tends to affect the body's sugar metabolism and means that a sugary substance called glycogen is deposited in the cells of the vaginal walls, and this tends to encourage the growth of thrush. This is certainly the case during pregnancy. For this reason, it is often suggested that taking the Pill predisposes women to it, though recent research conducted with the modern, low-dose Pills has found that thrush is not any more common among Pill users. Past studies showed a link between the Pill and thrush, but these were the old, high-dose Pills which contained high levels of oestrogen and which are not normally in use any more. There is no evidence to link the modern contraceptive pill with thrush, although some women swear that they get thrush when they go on the Pill and that the problem goes away when they come off it.

Other women find that their thrush flares up regularly once a month just before and during their period, only to retreat when the bleeding has stopped.

Many women notice that thrush flares up after they have had sex, and this often happens at the beginning of a new relationship when a woman has not had sex for some time. It is possible that this can be caused by the penis carrying thrush spores from the skin, especially near the anus, into the vagina where it can multiply in the warm, moist interior. More probable, however, is that the engorgement of tissues and secretions released during sexual excitement and intercourse provide a perfect breeding ground for thrush.

During sex, small amounts of fungus will be spread around

and rubbed into the vaginal tissues. Any small abrasions to the vaginal wall may also help the thrush to invade deeper into the tissues. It is not known whether the thrush fungus lives only on the surface of the vaginal wall, or whether it goes deeper into the cells when it flares up and causes a problem.

The hormonal changes which take place in pregnancy can also cause thrush, and many a woman finds that she gets thrush for the first time when pregnant, and the infection can prove much more difficult to treat while she is pregnant. It is also known that the pregnant woman's immune system seems to work less effectively; this may partly be because the immune system is slightly suppressed to enable the mother to carry a foreign being in her womb without being rejected, as happens to other foreign bodies or tissues, making transplants so difficult.

The menopause usually heralds the end of thrush, as the level of oestrogen decreases, unless you are on HRT. However, women undergoing the menopause may have swings in hormone levels which make them particularly prone to thrush.

It is not common knowledge that men can carry thrush on their penis, especially if they have not been circumcised, and can continue to reinfect their partner. Some doctors therefore think it's important that both the woman and her sexual partner should be treated. If the man is affected, usually a rash will appear on the skin quite quickly after he has been in contact with thrush, as soon as three hours after having sex with a woman who has a thrush attack.

However, it's probably quite rare for the man to be causing the problem; it's really a joint problem, because the woman has to be susceptible. Occasionally it can be found that the man is suffering from diabetes, and the sugary urine is encouraging the growth of thrush, and this keeps being passed on to the woman, so if a woman has recurrent thrush, it might be suggested that her partner is looked at too.

The use of a contraceptive cap, sponge or tampons can also keep reintroducing thrush into the vagina. IUDs have a thread which hangs down into the vagina and may provide a breeding ground for thrush, and so a change in contraceptive might be desirable.

The cap can obviously reintroduce thrush, so some doctors recommend that the cap is sterilised in Milton or infant feeding bottle sterilising tablets from time to time. This can perish the rubber, so you need to check your cap and have it replaced regularly.

Tampons can carry thrush from the skin surface into the vagina, and also tend to irritate the vaginal wall, especially when used at the end of a period, also helping thrush to get a hold.

Some women find that contraceptive creams, foams, gels and pessaries upset the normal acid/alkaline balance of the vagina and lead to a full-blown thrush attack.

One of the other main culprits is the use of nylon underwear, tights and tight-fitting trousers. These prevent air from circulating around the woman's genitals and create exactly the warm, damp conditions in which thrush thrives. Tight, hard trousers such as jeans can also chafe the skin, making it sore and worsening the situation.

Soaps, bubble baths, and other toiletries used on the vaginal area can kill off the protective bacteria and make a woman liable to thrush. If you are prone to thrush, you should never use soap on your genitals and avoid using bath salts, bubble baths and other chemicals on the skin. Hot water in the bath may also cause thrush to flare up, as it can encourage rapid growth of the fungus. Don't use the same flannel without washing on a hot wash and take care to clean your towels regularly, as this really is one infection which can linger on towels, especially in warm, damp bathrooms.

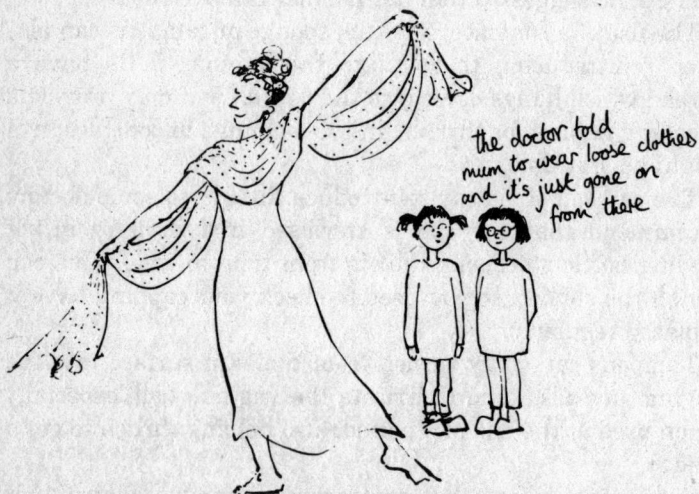

the doctor told mum to wear loose clothes and it's just gone on from there

Diet

Recently there has been a lot of talk about whether what you eat can predispose you to thrush.

There is certainly evidence that a 'junk food' diet containing lots of sugars, carbohydrates and not much fibre can predispose you to thrush. Long term, a diet like this will weaken your general health and your immune system. However,

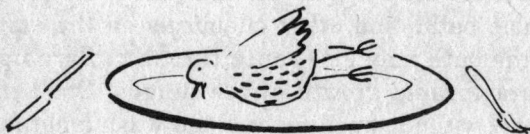

eating a lot of sugary substances can also trigger an attack of thrush.

There is a theory that avoiding foods with yeast will help avoid thrush, but this is controversial. More of this on page 131.

It is now thought that recurrent thrush may also be due to a defect in the woman's immune system which makes her prone to this infection. Or it may be that the woman has a specific allergy to a protein contained in the fungus which causes thrush, making her react with inflammation and itching to a level of thrush which most women would be able to tolerate without symptoms. Studies on thrush are difficult, because it is known that some women carry a detectable level of fungus but do not have symptoms, whereas others have a small amount of thrush but have severe symptoms.

Dr Angela Robinson at UCH GUM clinic says that it is difficult to carry out meaningful research into the causes and cures of recurrent thrush when the fungus is present normally and women have differing levels of sensitivity.

Women who react to low levels of fungus are often those who have other allergic problems, such as asthma and eczema. Marie had been plagued with thrush all her life. She had suffered from attacks of thrush regularly from her late teens. She tried her GP, a family planning clinic, a GUM clinic, but whatever she did, it kept coming back. The start of a new sexual relationship would often cause the thrush to flare up, causing inevitable problems. When she married, thrush flared up on her honeymoon, and she had thrush in her three pregnancies.

Swabs showed that she did indeed have thrush, but it was not always present in large amounts. As soon as she wore a pair of tights or jeans, the itching and soreness became unbearable. Every course of antibiotics caused an instant flare-up. Marie eats live yogurt, wears loose clothes, and always has a tube of anti-fungal cream with her. From time to time she uses pessaries to clear it up.

Doctors do not fully understand how it is that thrush gets a hold. One theory is that when thrush flares up, the fungus has changed from the form in which it simply divides by budding into the form in which it puts out long tentacles, called mycelae, which may grow down into the vaginal wall. This may mean that parts of the fungus actually invade the cells, and thus resist the action of anti-fungal creams and pessaries which work only on the outside. Then, when the fungicide is discontinued, the thrush flares up again.

Thrush and breast-feeding

It is not commonly known that thrush can live on the nipples and in the mouth of a new baby, and can go unrecognised, causing painful feeding for the mother and baby.

Thrush can be difficult to spot because sore nipples are not uncommon in the newly breast-feeding mother, and women don't realise that breast-feeding should never be really painful. Most sore nipples are caused by the baby not opening its mouth wide enough and latching on properly. A baby feeding with a small, pursed up mouth, as bottle-feeding babies do, will be tugging on the nipple and making it extremely sore. If this is the case, the nipples often look squashed when the baby comes off the breast, and the nipples can become blistered or even cracked. Many mothers give up breast-feeding for this reason.

Thrush, however, can grow on the nipples, making them red and sore even when the baby is feeding well. It can be difficult to spot, because mothers may mistake the redness for soreness caused by the baby's sucking, and white bits of fungus on the nipple can be mistaken for milk. If you are prone to thrush, and have vaginal thrush, the baby can pick this up during the birth and thrush can live in the baby's mouth. Again, this can be difficult to spot, as the white fungus can look like curds of milk.

Another problem is that the thrush can go through the

baby's gut and cause nappy rash, as the warm, damp nappy provides an ideal breeding ground. A thrush nappy rash has a distinctive look to the experienced eye: it is very red and blotchy, the skin is often raised and it is very itchy.

Mothers who have had courses of antibiotics for postnatal infections – perhaps an infected Caesarian scar or stitches to the perineum to repair a tear or episiotomy – are also particularly vulnerable to thrush, on the nipples as well as in the vagina.

Not all doctors, unfortunately, think of thrush on the nipples or are skilled at spotting it. Cressida had her first baby and was determined to breast-feed. Very soon her nipples became incredibly red and sore. She displayed them to the midwife, the health visitor, and the doctor, but no one recognised thrush. She was given help in trying to latch the baby on and was told that the baby was feeding well. The baby however appeared irritable, didn't sleep well and had a terrible nappy rash.

At nine weeks a breast-feeding specialist finally diagnosed thrush. The baby had thrush in her mouth and down her oesophagus, the tube which carries food down to the stomach. No wonder feeding had sometimes been uncomfortable for her, too. Cressida was given drops for the baby's mouth, cream for her nipples and the baby's bottom, and within twenty-four hours mother and baby were feeding and sleeping happily.

Don't scratch the itch!
No matter how much it itches, even if it's driving you mad, always resist scratching the vulval area. If you scratch the delicate skin, you will make it more inflamed, and this will create a better environment for the yeast to grow, so scratching – or rubbing – your vulva actually encourages the growth of thrush. If you break the skin, you may allow the fungus to penetrate deeper into the tissues, thus making it harder to

destroy. Scratching offers only a temporary relief, and will make the itching worse in the long term.

Occasionally doctors see women who have scratched the area so badly that they are red and scarred, and bleeding. This is quite rare – probably only about 1% of women who seek help for thrush – but you should always seek help before you get to this point!

HOW TO TREAT IT

If you think you have thrush, it is best to check by having a swab taken by your GP. If you have had thrush before and are sure you recognise the symptoms, this may not be necessary, but if you have recurrent thrush it is worth checking from time to time. Occasionally thrush can be mistaken for or mask another infection which might be more serious, such as bacterial vaginosis (usually caused by gardnerella) or chlamydia, so it is worth checking.

When a swab is taken it may be possible to have the result straight away. The discharge can be looked at under the microscope to see if the thrush spores and filaments are there. Moreover, a new accurate diagnostic test for thrush has been developed which can give a result in minutes. Vaginal swabs are taken and a drop of fluid is placed on a card slide which has been coated with antibodies to candida. If the cells clump together, the test is positive. Cultures can be grown, to make sure, but this takes a few days and you will have to wait for the results.

What drugs are available?
The standard treatment for vaginal thrush is anti-fungal creams and pessaries. The cream is applied externally to soothe itching, and the pessary is inserted into the vagina, usually at night.

Most anti-fungal agents don't actually kill the fungus, but prevent it from spreading or growing. One of the most popular anti-fungal agents, **clotrimazole** (sold as **Canesten**) acts by preventing the fungus from making a substance called ergosterol, necessary for making new cell walls.

The oldest anti-fungal agent in use is an antibiotic called **nystatin**, which is sold as **Nystan** cream and pessaries. Nystatin is bright yellow, and the pessaries and cream tend to stain your underwear, so are now rather unpopular. Nystatin can also be taken by mouth, usually as a course of pills to be taken four times a day for two weeks, to clear candida from the bowel. This is sometimes advised in cases of recurrent thrush or where thrush is present in the mouth.

Clotrimazole (**Canesten**) comes as pessaries and cream. The 10% cream is suitable for treating vaginal thrush, and this is now available off prescription. But beware: a recent survey showed that when women went into a pharmacy and asked for cream for thrush, a majority gave them **Canesten 1%**. This is intended for treating external fungal infections such as athlete's foot and is not effective against vaginal thrush.

Clotrimazole is white and non-waxy; the pessaries have a slightly crumbly, chalky texture, and most women prefer it to nystatin. The cream comes in a white and red tube and also a white and blue tube in which it also contains a steroid, hydrocortisone, which helps reduce itching and inflammation and is especially helpful where the woman seems to have an allergic reaction to the fungus. The steroid version is only available on prescription.

Econazole (sold as **Ecostatin**, **Gyno-Pevaryl**, **Pevaryl**) is another anti-fungal agent which comes as creams and pessaries.

Femstat is an anti-fungal cream derived from **butoconizole**, which has recently been approved in the US and has fewer side-effects than others.

Miconazole (Monistat, Gyno-Daktarin) comes in pessaries, coated tampons, cream or gel and also in tablet form. Side-effects are rare but can include skin irritation, nausea and vomiting.

Recently another group of drugs, **ketoconazole, fluconazole**, and **itraconazole**, have become available. These can be taken as one tablet by mouth and are systemic drugs, going through the whole body and destroying thrush on the skin. These are usually only prescribed where creams and pessaries have failed to solve the problem, as they can have side-effects. The fact that they are taken by mouth is a great boon for many women. 'After years of messing around with gungy creams and pessaries, it was bliss. I took one tablet at bedtime and hey presto! the symptoms had completely gone within a couple of days.'

DO THE DRUGS HAVE SIDE-EFFECTS?
Nystatin is a drug which has been in use for a long time and seems to have very few side-effects. Occasionally it seems to cause nausea and vomiting.

While **fluconazole (Diflucan)** seems to be very safe, there are reports that very rarely it may cause liver problems. The first drug of this kind to be introduced, called **ketoconazole**, is now rarely used because of some adverse drug reactions. It has caused hepatitis, which may not be reversible, causing liver failure and resulting in a very few deaths. Women with persistent recurrent thrush, who may take the drug fluconazole regularly, may need to have their liver function monitored. Another drug from the same group which is sometimes prescribed is **itraconazole (Sporanox)**.

One study of women with chronic or recurrent thrush showed **itraconazole** to be very effective in clearing up and preventing symptoms. The women took a dose of 200mg of itraconazole for three days; twelve of the twenty-one patients were cured. The remaining nine repeated the treatment, and they too were cured. The women were then given 200mg of itraconazole once a month for six months to try to prevent the condition recurring. Only one woman had a relapse in the second month, but after taking one 200mg tablet she was cured for the rest of the study period. Three months after the end of the treatment, 85% of the women remained cured.

Although these two drugs, fluconazole and itraconazole, seem very safe, thrush is not a life-threatening condition and therefore some women are reluctant to take a powerful drug which might have some small risk attached. Doctors do not like to prescribe it as a first choice because of this small risk. They are worried that resistance might develop, which would make fluconazole a less useful drug for treating the really severe thrush problems which can be life-threatening in cancer patients and AIDS sufferers. However, for some women who have tried everything else and are so desperate to get rid of their thrush, the small risk is acceptable.

Fluconazole has not yet been passed as safe to take during pregnancy, and should be avoided by those with liver or kidney disease.

An old remedy for thrush is **gentian violet**. This dark purple liquid used to be available from chemists and was used to treat fungal infections of the skin or vagina. It was not uncommon for women to be painted inside and out with it:

'I went into hospital for a D and C and they said my vagina was absolutely stuffed with thrush. It's true I'd suffered from thrush on and off for years and I'd just learned to live with it. They painted me with gentian violet and it worked; the thrush vanished and never came back. However, it did cause problems. All my clothes got stained with it for weeks afterwards and the first time I made love, my husband's penis came out blue!'

Women could paint gentian violet on their vulva to relieve external itching, but introducing it into the vagina is more tricky. Soaking a tampon in the solution and putting this in is one way. Recently, however, it's been shown that in large quantities gentian violet can be carcinogenic, or cancer-causing, so pharmacists and doctors now prescribe it with some reluctance. If all else has failed, however, one treatment is unlikely to cause any harm but women need to be aware of this and accept responsibility.

Women occasionally react to the creams and pessaries with soreness and irritation of the skin. This is then mistaken for the thrush continuing, and so the woman keeps using the creams and provokes more irritation. This happened to Dawn. 'It was driving me mad. You can buy the cream over the counter, so I kept doing this, applying it twice a day and putting it on a tampon to insert into my vagina. Finally I went back to my GP in desperation, she did a swab, and it came back clear. She suggested that the cream might be causing the problem and advised me not to use it for a while to see what happened. The itching cleared up instantly.'

In some cases it may be the anti-fungal agent the woman reacts to, in some cases the cream base. It is worth trying different formulations to see if there is one which is best for you.

PROBLEMS WITH PESSARIES

Using the pessaries can be tricky. Most of them come with a plastic applicator to help you insert the pessary high into the vagina, but many women find it easier and more comfortable to insert them by hand. Push them up into the vagina as high as you can; don't worry, there's no way you can push them up into the womb (uterus) or cause yourself any harm! It's best to do it last thing at night as you go to bed, to give them time to work. During the day they tend to descend the vagina, and lumps of pessary may come out.

Some of the pessaries, such as Canesten, tend to have a chalky, lumpy texture; they can be hard and scratch the vaginal wall. Others have a softer, waxier consistency. The sensation of bits of pessary leaking out over the next twenty-four hours is not a pleasant one, and some women hate using them. Pessaries with a waxy texture may be preferable.

Usually one pessary is enough, combined with the cream. However, in cases of persistent thrush, you may be given a course of pessaries to use in a three to six day course. Some doctors suggest you use a pessary once a fortnight for some time to see if you can stop the thrush recurring.

Other treatments

Anti-fungal agents alone may not work the trick, because the thrush fungus is normally carried on the skin and if the woman is susceptible, the symptoms may well simply come back again. In cases of stubborn and persistent thrush, women often try other remedies.

Sometimes a douche of **povidone iodine**, sold as **Betadene** can help. Douches are more popular in France and in the States than here, but while it is messy, it may work. The doctor may prescribe you one but you should be screened for other infections first. Lie in an empty bath and gently squeeze the fluid into your vagina. Make sure you follow the instructions, as too much pressure could be damaging and force the fluid into your womb. Never douche while pregnant or just before, during or after a period, as the cervix (neck of the womb) is slightly open at these times. The main risk is causing more serious infections in the womb or tubes.

Another treatment which helps is **bathing in salt water**. This alleviates the itching and also helps kill off the fungus. Don't use too much salt or it will sting; one teaspoon of salt per pint of water is about right. You can also use vinegar – one tablespoon of vinegar to a pint of warm water.

Live natural yogurt has often been suggested as another remedy. This is because the yogurt contains natural bacteria which are harmless and which tend to create an environment hostile to the fungus. You should use unsweetened, live

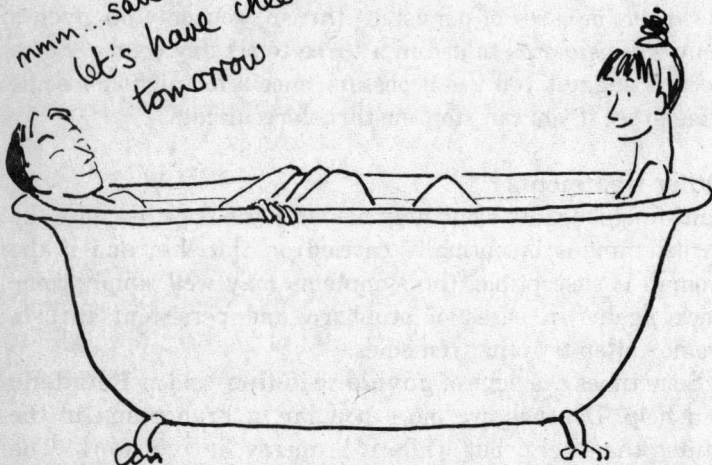

mmm...salt and vinegar bath – let's have cheese and onion tomorrow

varieties containing the bacterium lactobacillus acidophilus. The theory is that if thrush is caused by a lack of the normal, healthy bacteria on the skin, that you can replace this with natural yogurt. This should be applied externally and you should also include it in your diet. Use of yogurt – especially cool out of the fridge – is very soothing to sore tissues and it does seem to work for some women. You can also soak a tampon in yogurt and insert it into the vagina or almost literally spoon it in.

'I used the yogurt treatment with some success but it is very messy. It's easier to use in the summer when you're not wearing a lot of clothes, otherwise your clothes all become damp and smell of yogurt and apart from not being very nice, I think damp clothes make the thrush worse.'

Garlic is another natural anti-fungal agent. Some recent research has demonstrated how effective it is as both a bacterial killer and fungicide. Research at the Boston University Medical Centre and Rhode Island Hospital found that freshly pressed garlic extract, even diluted to one part in 250, proved effective against all the organisms in the laboratory study, including drug-resistant strains of bacteria.

The active ingredient in garlic is allicin, which is also responsible for its highly pungent smell. Of course, it is not clear how much of the substance allicin reaches the site of infection when it is eaten and digested, but applied externally to the skin, it is highly effective, and thus is a good way of beating thrush.

If you like garlic, use a lot of it in your food. You can also eat garlic on its own if you can bear it – and if the people around you can. If you or they can't stand it, you can buy special garlic capsules which don't smell from a health food shop or some chemists.

An extreme remedy is to take a clove of garlic, thread it with strong thread, and insert it into your vagina like a tampon. Leave it in overnight, and put a new one in the next night if necessary. Women say this works, but it does have the effect that the garlic seems to invade every pore of your body and you smell of it everywhere. Most people who've tried it once say never again, and it's a measure of the desperation some women feel that they're willing to try it at all!

Olive oil contains a substance called oleic acid which also helps prevent the thrush from changing into its aggressive form. You need to eat the olive oil raw, in salad dressing, rather than fried. Rubbing it on your vulva may also help.

HOW TO PREVENT IT

Once you have had thrush, it has a horrible habit of coming back to haunt you again and again. So once you've treated one

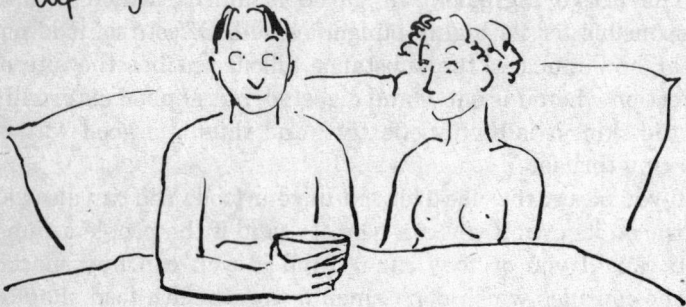

Let me just check that I've got this right - you want me to dip my penis in this live yoghurt and garlic THEN have sex...

attack, the next question is inevitably how to prevent it happening again?

Avoid antibiotics

Try to do without antibiotics if at all possible. Obviously if you have a serious infection, such as acute cystitis, pneumonia, severe tonsillitis or septicaemia, no one is going to suggest that you should do without. In these circumstances antibiotics can be life-savers.

However, there is a tendency for all of us to take antibiotics too soon, and without any real evidence that they are needed. The vast majority of colds and flus, sore throats and other infections are caused by viruses. These will clear up in their own time, usually within a week, just as well whether or not you take antibiotics. Indeed, antibiotics will sometimes make things worse by killing off the protective bacteria in our bodies

74

and allowing harmful ones resistant to that antibiotic to flourish.

Doctors often feel under pressure to prescribe something to alleviate people's symptoms, and we tend to expect the doctor to help. In our modern, stressful lives we don't want to give ourselves two days off work or in bed to enable our bodies to rest and combat the infection; we want to battle on regardless. So we dose ourselves with over-the-counter medicines to suppress the symptoms and take antibiotics. It is not uncommon for people to take several courses of antibiotics a year, none of them strictly necessary.

If you really do have to take an antibiotic, and you are prone to thrush, then ask your doctor to provide an antifungal pessary and cream to use at the same time. This may prevent a flare-up of thrush. You may need to use it for a while after you've stopped taking the tablets, as it takes a while for the protective bacteria to regrow on the skin and for your body's defences to get back to normal.

Washing your clothes
Thrush can live on your clothes, especially your underwear, and on towels, and represent a constant source of reinfection, so you need to pay attention to how you wash them.

The thrush fungus can survive at quite high temperatures, and you need to wash your towels and underwear at over 80° C if you want to kill it completely. You can wash most towels – especially white ones – at this temperature, but this may be problematic for delicate underwear. White cotton pants, however, can be washed at high temperatures.

If you can't wash everything at such heat, then ironing the crotch area of pants and trousers with a hot iron can also kill off any traces of the fungus.

Keeping towels in a damp, warm place may well enable the fungus to thrive, so make sure your bathroom is well aired and not damp, and dry your towels on a heated towel rail or radiator, and let the air get at them too if possible. If you are sharing a flat, take care with one another's towels as the infection can be spread from one person to another in this way.

Clothing

If you wear tight nylon clothing such as nylon pants, tights, leggings, leotards and tight jeans, you will keep the vaginal area moist, damp and airless, providing the ideal environment for thrush to grow. Thrush cases became far more common when tights overtook stockings in popularity, and the recent fashion for tight Lycra leggings and leotards has also led to many women experiencing their first attack of thrush.

If these are your favourite clothes, you may feel daunted at having to buy a new wardrobe and finding a new look for yourself. However, if you get rid of the thrush fungus once and for all, it will be worth it.

Our damp, cold English climate doesn't make it any easier either. Summer is with us at best for only three months of the year, and the rest of the time the main problem is how to keep warm. It may seem easy to wear skirts or dresses with no tights and cotton pants in the summer, or even be really daring and wear a long summery skirt with no pants, but how is one to manage in the cold spring, autumn and winter months?

Wearing lots of loose layers is an excellent way to keep warm. Buy natural fibres which allow the skin to breathe; these are also usually warmer than artificial ones. You can still wear trousers; but loose-fitting, baggy ones with plenty of room at the crotch, and again, buy natural fibres with a high cotton content if possible.

If you like stockings, wear these rather than tights. Some women – and their partners – find stockings really sexy and not fiddly once they get used to them. Other women, however, used to the ease of putting on tights, and unused to the sensation of the bare gap at the top of their legs, find stockings uncomfortable. Others associate them too much with strippers and sexy adverts and don't feel that they are right for them. If you feel like this, then there are brands of 'open gusset' or crotchless tights on the market. One of the most widely available is 'Pretty Cool' by Pretty Polly, which comes in a range of standard shades.

Soaps, bubble baths and deodorants

As with cystitis, you should avoid highly perfumed soaps, bubble baths and bath salts which irritate the skin and may cause a flare-up of thrush. If you have thrush, never use soap in the vulval or vaginal area, as this kills off the protective bacteria on the skin and allows the thrush fungus to take hold. You can clean the area perfectly adequately with your hand and warm water. Very hot water may also cause the area to be inflamed, kill protective bacteria and lead to a flare-up of thrush.

You should also avoid vaginal deodorants and fresheners like the plague. Again, these kill off the protective bacteria and make infection with thrush or other harmful organisms much more likely. There is no reason at all to think that the vaginal area is unpleasant or smelly; if it is, it's a sign that there may be something wrong. Many men find the natural smell of the vagina exciting, so there's no need at all to mask it with artificial scents.

Stress and feeling 'run down'

There is no doubt at all that thrush tends to thrive when we are feeling stressed, run down and unwell. When the body's natural defences are low, that's when thrush gets a hold and starts causing trouble.

Obviously it's far easier to say 'avoid stress' than it is actually to rearrange your life so as to make things easier for yourself, and for many women, the notion may seem impossible. Perhaps top of the list are young working mothers. Starting the day before six, dressing, feeding, and organising the children and getting them to the child-minder, nursery or school before arriving at work means that you feel you've put in a whole day before you even start work. Then there's the rush after work, the round of after-school activities, cooking one supper for the children and another for your partner when he comes home, getting them into bed, clearing up, tidying, answering letters and paying bills, and then, finally, bed, where all too often women feel under pressure to have sex with eager husbands! It's all too much, and the symptoms soon begin – chronic fatigue, colds that won't go away, eye, ear or sinus infections, cystitis, thrush and a whole host of other miseries all following one after another. 'I never feel well,' complain these women. They are miserable, so the children are miserable and demanding, their partner is miserable, and so on.

What can you do? You can't give the children away. You need the money from work. Women tend to soldier on until something gives, they get really ill, help is called in, and suddenly the woman gives up work or does something radical. Sometimes these disasters make the whole family re-evaluate things; but if you're stressed out already, why not act before it's too late? Turn to page 120 for tips on healthy living and how to take control before things take control of you.

The 'yeast connection' – is it a myth?

A great deal has been written about 'chronic candidiasis', a condition characterised by severe lethargy, depression, poor memory, headache, abdominal discomfort and bloating, together with vaginal thrush infections. The theory is that when these symptoms develop, the person's gut is overgrown by candida, and that this causes the body to develop an allergy to yeast substances in the environment. The cure is oral nystatin tablets and creams and pessaries to cure the vaginal candida, together with a very strict, low-carbohydrate, low-sugar, no-yeast diet.

There is no real evidence that this condition exists and that the diet works. A great deal of money has been made by doctors and authors who insist that all your problems will be cured if you only take the tablets and follow the diet. Unfortunately, it's not as simple as that. Stress and chronic fatigue are real twentieth-century diseases; then there is the 'post viral fatigue syndrome', known as 'yuppy flu', and the debilitating ME or myalgic encephalitis, which is also the subject of some controversy. Depression and mental problems are also part of the picture, especially for people who, because of the economic situation, are caught in boring, dead-end jobs, or worse, are unemployed.

At the present time people who are in work seem to be overworked, stressed out, doing several people's jobs at the same time and never being able to take time off. On the other hand there are those with no work and no prospects of getting work. It can't go on. Sooner or later people's physical and mental health suffers. You can't work on overtime all the time without your body or your mind ultimately calling a halt.

The proponents of the candida connection provide questionnaires asking things like, 'Do you have attacks of anxiety or crying?' 'Do you have heartburn or indigestion?' Symptoms such as an inability to make decisions, feeling 'spacy' or 'unreal' feature on the list. There are very few of us who don't sometimes experience these conditions. Almost all of us have taken antibiotics sometime in the not so distant past and many will have had vaginal irritation or discharge. By the time you've finished filling in the questionnaire you're almost bound to end up with a high probability that you've got 'chronic candidiasis'.

Doctors who support this hypothesis link a variety of other symptoms with candidiasis. These include premenstrual tension, urticaria, even mitral valve prolapse, a minor irregularity in the closing of a heart valve which occurs in healthy people and has no medical significance. These doctors argue that candida may weaken the person's immune system, rather than being the symptom of a weakened immune system. But since candida frequently becomes a problem in people who have AIDS or who have had their immune systems suppressed with radiotherapy, chemotherapy or drugs to prevent rejection of transplanted organs, it seems fairly obvious that candida is the symptom rather than the cause. So, take a break and cure your thrush. If you want to try the anti-candida diet, turn to page 130.

CHAPTER 3

Could It Be
Something Else?

OTHER INFECTIONS SOMETIMES MISTAKEN FOR THRUSH AND CYSTITIS

If you've already had thrush and cystitis, then you can be fairly sure of recognising them accurately again if you have a repeat infection. But this isn't always so. If you've had thrush and start itching again, you may immediately think 'thrush' and slap on the anti-fungal cream, when in fact the cause is something else – the treatment won't work. Or you may go to the doctor for antibiotics with the first twinge of what you think is cystitis only to find it's something else and you've taken the antibiotics for nothing.

So what else could it be? If you have any itching, discharge or pain in the lower regions, these are some of the options. Although they're far less likely than the two common offenders above, the fact that there can be confusion and that some of these infections or infestations can have serious consequences shows the importance of having a proper medical check if you have any infection which won't go away.

Bacterial vaginosis
This is one of the commonest causes of a vaginal discharge in sexually active women, with the exception of thrush, and it is

the condition most commonly confused with thrush. It usually causes soreness and a yellow or grey-white discharge. The main difference to thrush is that it usually smells and thrush tends to be more itchy.

The most common organism found in bacterial vaginosis – B.V., as it is now commonly known – is gardnerella vaginalis. B.V. seldom clears up without treatment, though it sometimes seems to disappear during a period, only to flare up again afterwards. The fishy smell is characteristic which can be quite powerful and is often noticed most during or after sex.

Marjorie had suffered from thrush many times over the years, so when the itching and discharge began she assumed that was what it was. 'I just bought the creams and treated myself as usual, and was surprised when it didn't go away.' Although she noticed the fishy smell, she didn't realise this was anything abnormal, and since she washed every morning and bathed at night, it never seemed overwhelming. 'Then I was working in the library on a hot afternoon, and someone said, "Can you smell something funny in here? It smells like fish." One woman turned round and sniffed in her shopping

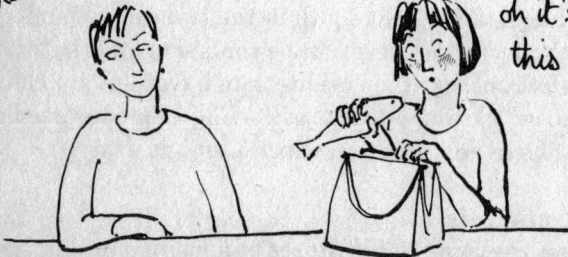

what's that strange smell?.. oh it's probably this silly me

bag, but I realised at once it was me. I rushed off to the GP that evening and he took a swab and found gardnerella which was an indicator that I had B.V.'

Jo found out that she had B.V. when she went for infertility tests at a London hospital. She had had a miscarriage and she and her boyfriend had been trying to conceive again for eighteen months. 'At an early appointment they did a vaginal examination and the doctor said it looked as if I had thrush. I'd had it before, and said so. He sent off the swab and it came back as gardnerella. I took a course of drugs which cured it, and two months later I was pregnant. I've often wondered if the infection hadn't been responsible for making the vagina hostile to sperm, and making it more difficult for me to get pregnant.'

It isn't known whether B.V. has this effect, but it *is* now known that it can precipitate premature labour in pregnant women. It's therefore very important to eliminate this organism before you get pregnant and to seek treatment if you have a discharge while you are.

TREATMENT

The drug used to treat it is usually a very powerful antibiotic called **metronidazole** (**Flagyl**). This is active against anaerobic bacteria (bacteria which survive and flourish in airless conditions) and protozoa (which cause trichomonas vaginalis, see below). Metronidazole can cause unpleasant side-effects, including nausea, a furred tongue and an unpleasant taste in the mouth, and should not be taken while pregnant, and with caution while breast-feeding. You should not drink alcohol while taking it; to do so may cause severe vomiting. Some women also get skin rashes and depression.

Metronidazole is usually taken as a course of tablets. It can also be taken as suppositories in the vagina or anus, or vaginal sponges impregnated with this drug have also been tried with success.

A relatively new treatment may be prescribed as an alternative, **clindamycin cream (Dalacin)**.

Pubic lice or crabs

Pubic lice – pediculosis pubis, to give them their proper name – are small insects looking a little like minute crabs. They are similar to head lice but live in the pubic region rather than on your head. Contracting pubic lice is no more shameful than your child catching head lice at school – it simply means that you've been in close contact with an infected person. You don't even need to have had sexual intercourse with them – an intimate hug in which your pubic hair comes into contact with someone else's is sufficient. Very occasionally they can be caught from infected bedding or towels, although they don't survive for very long once off the human body.

The symptoms are a maddening itch, often at its worst in the middle of the night. The itching is caused by a substance excreted into the skin by the insect when it bites. The insect, like a mosquito, sucks small quantities of blood from inside the pubic hair follicles. The lice lay eggs which hatch out in a few days and carry on biting, sucking blood and laying more eggs, till the infestation reaches unbearable proportions.

Pubic lice are hard to spot at first: they measure only about one to two millimetres in diameter. The eggs or nits are even smaller, only about half a millimetre in diameter. The eggs are glued to the hairs, usually near the base, and appear grey when full and pearly white after the lice have hatched out. If you have a heavy infestation, the tiny whitish specks may well become easily visible.

TREATMENT

Don't be tempted to shave off the pubic hair – you may well just scratch the skin, making the soreness and itching worse. Crabs can easily be treated by the same insecticides used to kill head lice – **malathion** and **carbaryl**. These are sold

84

under a variety of brand names including **Full Marks**, and **Lyclear**. You can buy preparations which act as a ten-minute shampoo or as lotions which can be left on overnight; these tend to leave some lasting protection against a new attack. Obviously your sexual partner or whoever you caught it from should be treated too (more of this in Chapter 4).

After treatment with the lotion or shampoo, you can remove the dead lice and some eggs with a nit comb, a very finely toothed comb. With some preparations you should repeat the treatment a few days alter.

You should also take the precaution of laundering your bedding, towels etc., in a hot (near boiling) wash. The lice will die within twenty-four hours of being deprived of the human host. The eggs take a week to ten days to hatch, so after two weeks away from all human contact all lice and nits will be dead. If you don't want to get your mattress cleaned, the simplest solution is therefore not to sleep on it for two weeks.

Occasionally the insecticides used to treat lice will cause itching and irritation, but this will usually clear up on its own in a few days.

Genital herpes
Genital herpes is caused by a virus similar to the one which causes cold sores around the mouth and lips, generally when you've got a cold or are run down. The cold sore virus is known as herpes simplex Type 1. Genital herpes is caused by herpes simplex Type 2, but Type 1 can cross over, from mouth to genitals during oral sex.

The usual way of catching genital herpes, however, is during sexual intercourse. Extremely painful blisters are characteristic of genital herpes. Fever, a general feeling of malaise, and tender lymph nodes can also be the first symptoms. Sometimes the painful blisters are hidden behind the labia (lips) or are so small you can't see them. Symptoms may include itching and a discharge, which can be mistaken for thrush. Inflammation and swelling around the vulval area or urethra can make it very painful and difficult to pee, so it is sometimes mistaken for cystitis.

Herpes is at its most infectious just before and during the time you have the blisters, so it is very important to avoid sex at this time. The blisters develop quickly into ulcers which form scabs and heal up. The problem with herpes is that it tends to recur again and again. Once infected, a woman harbours the virus, and it can pop up again, just like a cold sore on the lip, when least expected.

No one is sure what triggers off a repeat attack. The virus can be reactivated following sexual intercourse which causes some damage to the delicate mucous membranes of the vulval area, hormonal disturbances, and emotional stress. Another vaginal infection can also trigger a recurrence. The virus can flare up when the woman is pregnant, and if this happens at the end of the pregnancy the baby may be delivered by a Caesarian section, as it can be harmed if it picks up the virus while passing down the birth canal. During an episode of herpes, the woman can pass it on to her sexual partner, so must avoid sex when this happens.

TREATMENT

Herpes, being a virus, does not respond to antibiotics, so cannot be 'cured'. In the first episode of herpes, a course of **acyclovir** – an antiviral agent – can shorten the length of time the blisters/ulcers are present. It is important to go to your doctor or a specialist clinic to find out for sure what the problem is and get some treatment. An attack can be relieved by **salt baths** or bathing the area with a salt solution (one teaspoon of salt to a pint of water; a stronger solution may sting). You can use ice packs to relieve the pain, and **witch hazel** will help dry out the sores. Other common-sense measures include keeping the vaginal area cool by wearing loose clothes and cotton pants, and avoiding nylon tights will help.

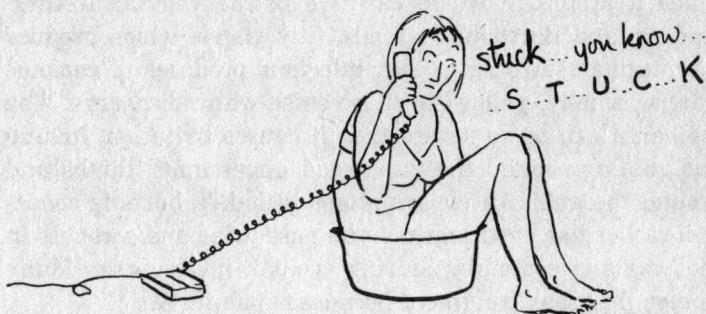

stuck... you know...
S...T...U...C...K

Milk compresses applied three to four times a day may help relieve the pain, and **lignocaine**, a local anaesthetic, can be used in severe cases. If the pain is really bad when you pee, you can try spraying the area with cold water from a plastic bottle with a spray top. Sitting in a bowl of cold water to urinate, or urinating in the bath, can help.

Because a connection between herpes Type 2 virus and cervical cancer has been suggested, it is usually recommended that you have regular cervical smears after herpes has been diagnosed.

Trichomonas vaginalis
'Trich', as it is popularly known, is a common vaginal infection usually passed on through sexual contact. Theoretically it can be picked up from damp towels and flannels or from a splash from an unflushed lavatory but this is highly unlikely. Swimming pools aren't a cause of contamination – as has been suggested – as the organism responsible dies very quickly when in contact with chlorine. Sometimes a low grade infection can flare up, especially just before a period.

Trichomonas vaginalis is a small microscopic organism called a protozoan which can live in the vagina, urethra, bladder, and Bartholin's glands, tiny glands which produce the vaginal secretions. The infection produces a copious, watery, smelly, yellowish or greenish-white discharge. The discharge can be so severe that it causes irritation, itching and chafing around the vulva and upper inner thighs and around the anus. Other symptoms include a burning sensation rather like cystitis when you pass urine and soreness in the vagina, especially during sexual intercourse. Many women first seek treatment because of painful sex.

About one woman out of five is carrying this organism without developing any symptoms, although it isn't a normal inhabitant of the vagina like thrush or of the gut like E. coli, the most common cause of cystitis. Even if the protozoa end up in the mouth or rectum during sex, they cannot survive there long enough to reinfect the vagina.

Although men can be infected and carry the organism, it survives only in the urethra and doesn't ascend any further. It can't live in the rectum or elsewhere on the man's body. A man will rarely get symptoms. If he does it will be some faint stinging on passing urine. So most men are not aware that they are infected. Since the man can immediately reinfect his female sexual partner, he should be treated along with the woman.

Trichomonas vaginalis can be detected if a vaginal swab is taken. It can also be detected when a cervical smear is taken, and in fact the presence of trich is one of the most common causes of an atypical cervical smear. Many cases of trichomonas come to light because of a routine smear test.

TREATMENT
The treatment for trich is the antibiotic **metronidazole**, (**Flagyl**), also used to treat bacterial vaginosis (see above). A single course will clear up the infection in 95% of cases.

Once you take the medicine, the itching, discharge and other symptoms should disappear within two or three days. However, it's very important to continue and finish the course of antibiotics and also to treat your sexual partner if you want to avoid a recurrence.

It is not uncommon for a thrush infection to mask an infection with trichomonas vaginalis, and the two infections sometimes go together. So it's always important to have a swab taken if your thrush doesn't seem to respond to anti-fungal drugs or if your discharge is unusually smelly.

Chlamydia

Chlamydia is now one of the commonest sexually transmitted diseases, although it has only been recognised fairly recently. The bacterium chlamydia trachomatis was probably, however, the most common cause of what is known as non-specific urethritis or NSU.

Chlamydia infects the vagina and cervix, and in women can be completely symptomless. Sometimes it causes a discharge, and pain when passing urine. Again, it is sometimes mistaken for early cystitis or for thrush.

In men, infection is usually followed by a discharge from the penis, but it can also be symptomless. This means that a man can infect a woman without his knowing it; she in turn may be unaware that she has it. If she does develop symptoms, this is usually up to four weeks after exposure to infection. Chlamydia is often diagnosed when a woman goes to be investigated for other gynaecological problems, and has a vaginal examination and swab.

As a woman it's very important to get treatment, because if it's not dealt with, chlamydia can ascend up from the vagina into the womb and the tubes and lead to pelvic inflammatory disease. This condition, PID, causes abdominal pain and can lead to damage and scarring of the tubes which can cause infertility or an ectopic (tubal) pregnancy. Of those women who get PID, 20% will have chronic pelvic pain, 15% will be infertile, and 5% will have an ectopic pregnancy.

An ectopic pregnancy is very dangerous, because if it's not detected early the pregnancy ruptures the tube and causes bleeding into the abdominal cavity. It is a medical emergency, and one of the worst aspects is that once ruptured, the tube is out of action for good. Bleeding can cause scarring and blockages of the other tube as well, and 50% of women who have an ectopic pregnancy will not conceive naturally again.

Research shows that after one episode of chlamydia, 20% of women will develop PID.

TREATMENT
Chlamydia is treated with one of the antibiotics in the tetracycline group. It usually needs a week of antibiotics or longer in the case of PID.

Vaginal warts
These are painless but itchy lumps of skin on the vaginal wall, the vulva, or the skin round the anus. They are caused by a virus. They sometimes appear singly, sometimes in large groups. They start off quite small but can grow uncomfortably large.

Vaginal warts are passed on during sex, though you can rarely pass one on from a wart on your hand if you touch your genital area. They can appear from two months to even years after exposure to infection. They tend to spread more quickly if you are pregnant. Vaginal warts are harmless, though there is a connection between them and cervical cancer, so if you have been infected you should have a regular cervical smear test, perhaps once a year initially.

TREATMENT
The treatment is to have the warts painlessly burned off with lasers, chemicals or cauterisation.

Bartholin's cysts or abscesses

The Bartholin's glands are situated on either side of the vagina and produce the secretions which keep the vagina moist and healthy. Occasionally one of these glands becomes infected with bacteria and an abscess can form. The gland swells, producing a discharge, and it can be very painful. Passing urine can also be very painful – like acute cystitis, so the symptoms are sometimes confused.

TREATMENT

The usual treatment is with antibiotics, though an abscess will need to be lanced and drained by a doctor if it doesn't clear up. If the entrance to the gland gets blocked and a cyst appears, a small operation may be needed to remove it.

Cervical polyps (see also Cervical erosion p. 97)

Polyps are small, fragile, almost always harmless growths which can appear in various different parts of the body. If you have a polyp on your cervix, it may get knocked during intercourse and bleed a little. It may also create a discharge, which can harbour bacteria and set off other infections.

TREATMENT

Polyps can easily be removed, either by twisting or freezing them off in a very minor operation for which anaesthetic should not be necessary. You may need to rest for a day or two to recover and there may be a little bleeding for three or four days until it has healed.

Cervical cancer

Cervical cancer is the second biggest killer of women after breast cancer, and this is terrible, because it is almost entirely preventable. If every sexually active woman had regular smear tests, the early signs of cervical cancer could nearly always be detected, and prompt treatment would mean that no one had to suffer the effects of this cancer.

Cervical cancer is a very slow cancer, and begins with the growth of pre-cancerous cells on the cervix. These then develop into cancerous cells, but remain restricted to the outer layer of the cervix. This is carcinoma in situ. These cells are detectable only with a microscope and are invisible to the eye, so can only be detected under a microscopic examination of suspect cells. There are no symptoms. Early cervical cancer normally progresses very slowly, and it may take ten years or more for the cancerous cells to invade the deeper cervical tissues, and longer still for them to spread elsewhere in the body.

Once the cancer has invaded the deeper cervical tissues, the symptoms may begin: irregular bleeding or spotting, especially after sexual intercourse, and from time to time an unpleasant, blood-tinged vaginal discharge. Even at this stage treatment can cure the cancer in the majority of cases.

Some women are known to be at higher risk of cervical cancer than others. These include women who started having sexual intercourse early, women who have had multiple sexual partners, and women who have had sexually transmitted infections such as herpes or genital warts. Cervical cancer is far less common in women who delayed having sex till later and who have had one or a few sexual partners. Changes in patterns of sexual behaviour therefore partly account for the recent increase in cervical cancer.

The risk of cervical cancer does also appear to be greater in women who have taken the pill for ten years or more. There does seem to be a direct link with the Pill itself, although it may be solely because the Pill has given women greater sexual freedom. Using the Pill also means that fewer women use the contraceptive cap or have partners who use the condom, and both of these tend to protect against cervical cancer. The recent upsurge in HIV infection and the threat of AIDS may reduce cervical cancer rates in the future, as people rely more on condoms and take more care in selecting their sexual partners.

Cervical smear tests are quick, more or less painless and you can read more about these on page 103.

Vaginitis

This is an irritation of the vagina which involves soreness, itching and dryness. It may occur after the menopause when levels of the female hormone oestrogen fall away, and the fluid produced by the vaginal walls which helps keep it moist and supple becomes scantier. Sexual intercourse can become painful and damage can be done to the delicate tissues; if there are small tears in the vaginal wall infections can more easily get a hold, and you may have a blood-tinged discharge which can be mistaken for something more serious. Occasionally the absence of lubrication can lead to an attack of cystitis.

TREATMENT

Vaginitis can usually easily be cured by applying creams containing oestrogen to the vaginal area. Using HRT, hormone replacement therapy, can also prevent or cure this condition. It's also very important that your sexual partner takes care to make sure that you are thoroughly aroused before attempting penetration, and you may also find using a colourless, odourless lubricating cream such as KY jelly is very helpful.

A forgotten tampon

Very occasionally you may forget to remove the last tampon of your period. This happens to nearly everyone at some time in their lives. After a few days you may notice a smelly discharge and some discomfort; usually this makes you inspect this region and you may either remember the tampon or discover the tampon threads. The tampon may be difficult to remove; you can always ask your GP to remove it or go to a casualty department. Don't worry, they'll have done this before and won't think you're an idiot.

Because of the danger of the toxic shock syndrome, in which a harmful bacterial infection can be set up on a tampon and which has even been known to cause death in a few instances, your doctor may well want to take a swab to see if you have a bacterial infection and may want to prescribe antibiotics. Toxic shock syndrome seemed to be linked to certain tampons containing deodorant substances or certain chemicals, so may now be less common. But if you discover a tampon has been left in and have an unpleasant discharge, it may be worth a quick visit to the doctor even if you've successfully removed it yourself.

Actinomyces

Actinomyces are filamentous fungi which may colonise the genital tract when a woman has an IUD (coil). The discharge may be mistaken for thrush. The fungus can grow on the IUD strings and ascend up into the womb, where it occasionally can cause pelvic inflammatory disease. If you have this problem, the first step is clearly to have the IUD removed. Actinomyces are sensitive to the antibiotics **penicillin** and **tetracycline**.

Streptococcus

The bacterium streptococcus is sometimes found causing irritation and a discharge in the vagina. It is most dangerous when a woman is pregnant, as it can set up a nasty infection in the baby when he or she passes down the birth canal during labour. It is easily treated with antibiotics.

Mycoplasma

This is an organism which can infect the vagina. There is some evidence to suggest that it may be a cause of pre-term labour.

Gonorrhoea

Known by a variety of names such as 'the clap' or 'a dose', this is the best known sexually transmitted disease. While some of the other infections listed above are often or almost always sexually transmitted, nothing has quite the same stigma as a case of gonorrhoea. However, no one should ever let shame put them off seeking help, as it is very easily treated and can have serious consequences if left untreated.

Gonorrhoea is an extremely contagious infection of the genital organs, caused by the bacteria Neisseria gonorrhoeae. The bacterium can only survive inside the body, so can only be passed by direct genital contact. Gonorrhoea can also be passed from one person to another through oral-genital sex and you can develop gonorrhoeal infections of the mouth and throat. If you have anal sex, you can also have an infection in the rectum, and this is often symptomless.

One problem with gonorrhoea is that 80% of women never develop any obvious symptoms. Some women can harbour gonorrhoea for a long time, transmitting it to their sexual partners, without knowing. In men, symptoms usually appear within three to seven days of contact with an infected person, although it can be as long as six weeks. About 10% of men never develop obvious symptoms, but in the great majority pain on urination or when they get an erection, and a discharge from the penis makes them seek immediate medical treatment. Most women realise they may have gonorrhoea when their current or previous sexual partner informs them that they have an infection.

Women infected with gonorrhoea can develop genital irritation, have a vaginal discharge or experience pain on urination. Some of these symptoms can of course be confused with the onset of thrush or cystitis. It's very important to seek help, because the infection can spread up into the womb and fallopian tubes and lead to infertility.

Gonorrhoea can often spread higher up because when a

woman has her period this creates the ideal breeding ground for the bacteria. Once the infection has spread into the fallopian tubes the woman may experience a fever, chills, abdominal tenderness, and pelvic pain after sexual intercourse.

TREATMENT

The treatment for gonorrhoea is an injection or single dose of antibiotics, and the drug of choice is still **penicillin**. If you are allergic to penicillin, **tetracycline** is sometimes given. **Spectinomycin** is an antibiotic developed specifically for gonorrhoea, and is usually given by intramuscular injection. These broad-spectrum antibiotics are likely to cause an attack of thrush, so ask for pessaries and cream to try to keep this at bay, and eat or apply live natural yogurt if you are prone to thrush.

Syphilis

Syphilis, that most dreaded of sexually transmitted diseases, is nowadays fortunately becoming very rare, so its inclusion here is mainly for completeness. People who suspect they have had a sexually transmitted disease will normally be tested for syphilis just to eliminate this possibility. Pregnant women are routinely tested, as undetected syphilis can have a devastating effect on the unborn baby. Apart from the fact that the disease is much rarer today, so that you're very unlikely to come across an infected partner, it's extremely unusual for anyone to develop syphilis without its being detected.

Syphilis is caused by an organism called a spirochete, treponema pallidum, to give it its Latin name. The first stage of syphilis is the development of the chancre or primary sore. It first appears as a painless ulcer somewhere on the genitals. This heals spontaneously in six to ten weeks. The chancre most commonly appears on the external genitals, especially in the man, but it can occur inside the vagina or even on the cervix, and thus go unnoticed; uncircumcised men can also miss it if it's under the foreskin. The chancre can also appear on the lips or inside the mouth or throat. The lymph glands are often also swollen at this stage. It can be difficult to distinguish from herpes but usually the ulcers in herpes are painful and there is more than one, unlike syphilis.

The organism then spreads silently through the bloodstream for a latent period, which can be quite short or quite long – often months. You then develop secondary syphilis, the symptoms of which are skin rashes, and sometimes a sore throat, loss of hair, and aching in bones and joints. During the first and second stages, the infected person is highly infectious to close genital contacts. If this goes undetected, the disease becomes latent again, and causes no symptoms, except that a pregnant woman can infect her child. It then emerges – sometimes as long as ten or fifteen years later – as tertiary syphilis, resulting in problems with the heart, brain, lungs, spinal cord, bone and skin. This terrible disease – general paralysis of the insane, as it used to be known – is almost unheard of today.

TREATMENT
Fortunately, syphilis today is highly curable if caught in the first and second stages. The antibiotic of choice is again **penicillin**.

Cervical erosion
The cervix is the neck of the womb. It feels and looks like a rounded knob, about 1–2 inches in diameter, which feels slightly hard and rubbery. In the centre is the cervical os, a tiny opening into the womb. Inside is the cervical canal. Through this blood is expelled during menstruation, sperm swim up from the vagina, and of course, during labour it stretches wide open to allow the baby's head and body to pass through.

The cervix secretes mucus, and this varies in texture according to the monthly menstrual cycle. In the middle of the month, when you are at your most fertile, it produces a copious, thin, transparent slippery mucus. Some women can recognise this and know that this is the time when they are most likely to conceive. At other times of the month the mucus is thicker and scantier.

Sometimes the cells of the outer part of the cervix are replaced by the kind of cells which normally lie in the cervical canal. The tissue looks inflamed and secretes more mucus, which can occasionally be bloodstained, especially after sexual intercourse. A cervical erosion usually occurs during puberty or after pregnancy because of the changing hormone levels, or in connection with taking the contraceptive pill.

A cervical erosion is harmless, but can be alarming, especially if you have a bloodstained discharge. It can also make you more prone to other infections such as thrush, because the extra discharge creates an ideal breeding ground for the thrush fungus. Cervical erosions are often detected during a routine pelvic examination or when a smear is taken.

TREATMENT
Erosions usually clear up on their own, and treatment is normally only suggested if symptoms persist and usually consists of cauterising, or burning off the cells responsible with a laser or electric cautery, a minor operation which is usually done without an anaesthetic.

CHAPTER 4

Getting Help:
Conventional and
Alternative Medicine

Where to get help

If you have cystitis or thrush, the first place you would
probably think of seeking advice is from your GP. However,
there are people who for many reasons may feel reluctant to
see their GP. Cystitis and thrush are too often linked with
your sex life, and you may not want your family doctor to
know about it. If, for example, you've been having a secret
affair, and you think your thrush or cystitis might be linked to
that, you might not want your GP to know. Or you might
want to be screened for any sexually transmitted infections at
the same time, and not want your GP to know that either.

Many people put off seeking advice and help because they
are ashamed of talking to their doctor. Usually there is no
reason for this, but it's very human and understandable. With
thrush, it may not be serious, but if you have an attack of
cystitis, then delaying can be dangerous. So you should
always seek help.

Often people don't seek help for completely the wrong
reason. Janey, aged fourteen, suffered from raging thrush for
months before telephoning a counsellor after hearing a
phone-in programme on the radio. The radio station provided

back-up counsellors off air, and she phoned in to ask what she had got. She thought that the thrush had been caused because she sometimes masturbated, and was afraid to go to her GP because she was ashamed of his knowing this. Once it was explained that this was nothing to do with it and that treatment could clear it up in a matter of days, she was intensely relieved.

If you can't face going to your GP, there is another, simple alternative: you can go to a GUM or Genito-urinary Medicine clinic (sometimes known as a Sexual Health Clinic), usually attached to your local hospital. These used to be called VD (venereal disease) clinics, then STD (sexually transmitted disease) clinics and have now been renamed GU or GUM clinics. You can just walk into a GU clinic without an appointment and be seen without a long delay. You can give a false name if you like and all your details are entirely confidential. In most GU clinics the staff are very helpful and friendly and the atmosphere is very different to that in many parts of the hospital.

Many women with thrush and cystitis are anxious about going to a GU clinic because they imagine they will be there with a lot of strange, furtive looking and promiscuous people. Nothing could be further from the truth. Quite a high proportion of people visiting a GU clinic do not have a sexually transmitted disease at all. At St Mary's, Paddington, for example, only about 15% of clients have a sexually transmitted disease, and the rest have other problems such as thrush, cystitis, gynaecological problems, sexual problems, and so on. One study showed that in 1989, 17% of all women attending GU clinics had thrush, sometimes on its own, sometimes with other infections. At St Mary's, about 5% have cystitis.

Many people use GU clinics to pop in for check-ups, for smear tests, and so on, perhaps partly because it's so easy to pop in without an appointment and get good, friendly treatment. Although this clinic may be a little unusual and at some

GU clinics there is probably a higher proportion of people with STDs, it will still be by no means the majority.

Sally visited a GU clinic for the first time when she was eighteen and had developed thrush. 'I sat there in this waiting room and I wanted to shout to everybody, "I'm not here for that, in fact, I'm a virgin, I haven't even had sex." But everyone else looked so normal that after a while I stopped worrying. I'm sure there were other people like me, in the same boat.'

Go prepared

Before you go to see the doctor, it always helps to make a short list of the questions you want to ask. This is because you get only a short time with the doctor, you will be examined and so on, and often you are given so much information that it's difficult to take it in. When you leave you may find that you are quite muddled and that you still don't know the answers to your basic questions.

It helps if you know as much about your condition as possible before talking to your doctor. Many doctors just assume their patients don't know much, and only provide detailed information when asked. People often don't like to ask in case they get answers they don't want, either. Questions like 'Do these pills have any side-effects?' may result in reassurance, but it may also result in an honest doctor telling you that all drugs have side-effects and that (very rarely) they can be serious.

If you know a little about your condition, this helps you to understand what the doctor is saying and understand your condition. Understanding your illness is the first step to overcoming it.

What the doctor will do

When you are seen by your GP or at a GU clinic you will first explain the problem to a doctor. Doctors at a GU clinic in

101

particular are used to dealing with people who have embarrassing ailments and are usually very relaxed and sympathetic.

The doctor will usually ask you exactly what symptoms you have. Try not to be too vague – saying 'It hurts down there' is not very helpful. Does 'down there' mean your bladder, your vagina, or somewhere else? With cystitis in particular, your doctor will probably ask you whether you've had it before, and if so when, how often, and how severely.

You will then normally be given a physical examination. If cystitis is suspected, the doctor will feel your tummy all over, including the area just above the pubic bone, and around each kidney. He or she should be able to detect any areas of tenderness, and in a slim person, any kidney swelling can usually be felt. The doctor will probably also take your blood pressure.

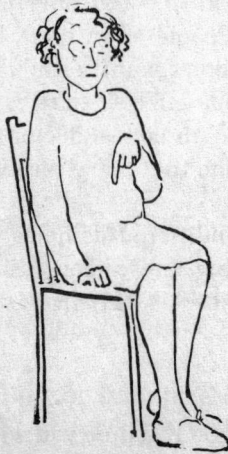

it hurts down here

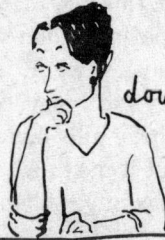

down there?

A urine sample will usually be taken, and a swab from your urinary tract and/or vagina. The doctor will often give you a proper internal examination and insert a speculum into the vagina to view the internal organs and look for any signs of discharge or disease.

Many women worry unnecessarily about having an internal examination. If sensitively done, it should not be at all painful and shouldn't really be even uncomfortable, especially if you relax. If you are very tense it will make it more difficult for the doctor to examine you, and usually mean he or she takes longer. It may actually be painful if you tense your muscles, so relaxing is quite important. Take some deep breaths and consciously relax yourself when lying on the couch, let your legs go floppy and try not to worry.

In order to view the walls of the vagina and the cervix, and to take a swab, the doctor will need to insert a speculum. This is a terrifying looking metal instrument which is slipped inside the vagina and then clamped open to hold the walls of the vagina apart. The doctor should then have a clear view of your cervix and vagina. If feasible a doctor will always warm the metal in warm water before inserting it and use a little KY jelly for lubrication. All the instruments will, of course, have been sterilised before use.

Having a vaginal examination is never pleasant, but it shouldn't hurt. You should never be left alone with a speculum, and make sure that the doctor or nurse doesn't 'pop out for a minute' in the middle of an examination. This happened to Claire, who found that she was then forgotten. 'I was quite comfortable, so I lay there for about fifteen minutes with the speculum clamped open inside me before it dawned on me that someone had forgotten me. Needless to say I couldn't attempt to get up, so I had to yell till someone came to rescue me!'

If there is a discharge, or signs of any irritation or infection, the doctor will take a swab for analysis. A cervical smear may be taken by using a special spatula or brush to scrape some cells from the cervix. Your cervix is not sensitive so you shouldn't feel this, but the top of the vagina *is* sensitive so women often feel the brush against it. This is not painful; some women find the sensation a little irritating and unpleasant, but it only lasts a few seconds. It is recommended that most women have a smear test every three years, but you may be advised to have one more frequently, if for some reason this might be necessary.

Once the speculum is removed, the doctor may then perform a bimanual examination to check the position of the internal organs. To do this, the doctor will slip one or two fingers inside the vagina and place the other hand above it on the abdomen. By pressing gently with the upper hand, the doctor will be able to feel the womb and ovaries and check that these are normal size, in the usual place, and whether the womb is mobile or held in place by scar tissue from a previous infection.

An examination and initial tests will most likely mean that you get a result very quickly and either have your fears put to rest or are able to leave the clinic with a diagnosis and prescription.

Contacting sexual partners

One service which all GU clinics offer is tracing sexual partners if it turns out that you have a sexually transmitted infection. If you have thrush or cystitis, then this won't apply, but if you have chlamydia or any of the other sexually transmitted infections listed in Chapter 4 then your partner will be contacted. This is always done discreetly and anonymously if you prefer.

If you have a sexually transmitted disease, then the possibility that you might have been infected with HIV may cross your mind. GU clinics will also do a blood test for HIV but you do need to think very carefully before you embark on this. If you were infected recently, a negative result may mean nothing, as it can take up to three months for the antibodies to become measurable, so you will need a re-test.

If you were to be tested positive, you would then have all the anxiety associated with this result, and might find that you could not get life insurance and were discriminated against in various ways. You should obviously practise safe sex, i.e. non-penetrative sex or sex with a condom, whether you are HIV positive or not, if you are not in a monogamous relationship. Discuss whether to have the test very carefully with the staff at the GU clinic, who will be very helpful in finding out what's best for you.

ALTERNATIVE THERAPIES

Let us assume that you have been through the conventional treadmill, and yet your problem keeps coming back. You've had antibiotic treatment for cystitis over and over again, but it keeps recurring. Or you can't get rid of the thrush, no matter how hard you try. You've had all the tests, and you know what the problem is and that it's not some other condition mimicking thrush and cystitis, and that there isn't some underlying health problem which is causing it. You may have got rather fed up with what conventional medicine can do, and want to try something different.

The alternative therapies actually have a very good track record in treating and preventing conditions such as thrush and cystitis. Indeed, many of the suggestions now made by people, including doctors, to treat stubborn and recurrent infections of thrush and cystitis originated with these therapies. In addition, when you go to see an alternative therapist you often receive a lot of care, attention, and sympathy which helps make you feel better in itself. Some treatments, such as an aromatherapy massage, are extremely pleasant and relaxing and may help your body to rest and recuperate naturally.

105

Increasingly doctors are recognising that a person's outlook and psychological approach has a large impact on illness. Although they have in the past been traditionally highly sceptical of alternative therapies, many are realising that, where conventional medicine doesn't help, alternative therapies may have much to offer. Cynically, one might say that these therapies may keep troublesome patients who keep coming back again and again with the same problem out of the surgery; but others are willing to accept that often these therapies achieve positive results.

When you go to see a practitioner of an alternative therapy, in particular acupuncture or homeopathy, the practitioner will spend a great deal of time talking to you, listening, and looking at you as a complete person, rather than only concentrating on your symptoms. A trained homeopath, for example, usually spends an hour and a half on the first consultation. Anne, a chronic cystitis sufferer, recalls: 'I went to see my doctor with cystitis and I got five minutes with him. I'd done a urine sample, and he just said, "Yes, it's cystitis, we'll send that off, and in the meantime just take these antibiotics." He did tell me to drink lots of fluids and to take some painkillers if it was too bad, but that was it. When I went to see the homeopath we spent an hour and a half talking about my cystitis, my general health, my relationship, everything. She was wonderfully sympathetic and seemed to understand for the first time what I was going through. She made a lot of suggestions which really helped. I came out of there for the first time feeling I was really getting somewhere.'

This book can obviously only give a quick introduction to the various therapies and suggest remedies which can be particularly helpful in treating cystitis or thrush.

Acupuncture

Acupuncture forms part of Chinese traditional medicine, which includes herbal medicine, exercise, massage and diet, and which has been in use for over 3000 years. Acupuncture uses fine needles to stimulate invisible lines of energy which run beneath the surface of the skin, changing the body's balance of energy and restoring a sick person to health. Moxibustion, the burning of herbs to stimulate the body's energy, is often used with acupuncture.

Like many alternative therapies, acupuncture is holistic, that is, it looks at the whole person rather than simply isolating symptoms and treating them.

Acupuncture is based on the idea that Qi (pronounced 'chee'), the vital energy of the body, flows through certain channels, creating a network throughout the whole body and linking all parts together. There are twelve main Qi channels, each connected to an internal organ and named after that organ. When a person is healthy the Qi flows smoothly through the channels, but if for some reason the flow is blocked or becomes very weak, illness occurs. The acupuncturist aims to correct the flow of Qi by inserting thin needles into particular points on the channels.

Acupuncture can be used as preventive medicine by correcting the energy before a serious illness can occur, and also to reverse illnesses by restoring the Qi.

The acupuncturist needs a detailed understanding of the patient's lifestyle, medical history, personality, work and so on before making a diagnosis. The pulse and tongue are examined to assess the body's energy and degree of illness. Not everyone responds to acupuncture, just as not everyone can be cured by conventional medicine. But, as many will testify, it can be highly effective.

Extensive research in China has shown that acupuncture is highly effective, and in the People's Republic of China traditional and modern medicine are equally used. In Western countries, this solid research has convinced many that acupuncture does work, and it is sometimes used for anaesthesia and pain relief in Western hospitals.

Acupuncture can be very effective in treating cystitis and vaginal discharge.

There is a code of practice laid down by the Department of Health which registered acupuncturists must follow. Information can be obtained from:

The Register of Traditional Chinese Medicine
   19 Trinity Road
   London N2 8JJ
   081–833 8431

or: The Council for Acupuncture (see page 145).

Aromatherapy

Aromatherapy has been described as the art and science of using essential plant oils as treatments. It is a holistic therapy, taking people's mind, body and spirit into account. Oils from plants have been used medicinally for thousands of years, and of course extracts of plant oils are used in modern medicines.

Essential oils are absorbed very rapidly through the skin, and the oils are used in massage, in baths, and in skin preparations or compresses. The essences can be diluted into a carrier oil such as pure olive oil, or in beeswax or other cream bases. A certain amount of the essential oil is also breathed in, and the scent has an effect on the mind and thus on the body. Part of the oil is also absorbed directly and rapidly into the bloodstream via the lungs. The effect of the oils, together with a soothing massage, a gentle soak in a bath and the contact with the therapist all combine to have a very beneficial effect.

AROMATHERAPY AND CYSTITIS

Aromatherapists recommend **Bergamot**, **Camomile**, **Eucalyptus**, **Garlic**, **Lavender** and **Sandalwood**. Bergamot is a powerful urinary antiseptic, and relieves depression and tension.

It can be used as an external wash and in the bath. Camomile calming and mildly diuretic, and can be taken in the form of camomile tea. Garlic can be taken in capsule form. Camomile and Bergamot can be combined in external washes which should be between ½ and 1% dilution of essential oil in boiled and cooled water. The opening of the urethra should be swabbed with this at frequent intervals and camomile tea should be drunk together with spring water or home-made lemon barley water. About six drops of Bergamot should be added to the bath.

A massage oil containing Bergamot, Lavender or Camomile can be used to massage the lower abdomen, and, if there is pain, a hot camomile compress may be useful. A whole body massage can soothe and relax the person and help relieve the depression which often goes with this condition.

Prompt treatment may stop an attack of cystitis before it takes hold, but antibiotics may be needed, and the aromatherapy can be continued together with antibiotic treatment if necessary.

AROMATHERAPY AND THRUSH

Aromatherapists recommend baths and local applications of **Lavender**, **Myrrh**, or **Ti-tree oil**. This treatment should continue for some time even after the initial symptoms seem to have cleared up.

It is important to consult a trained aromatherapist who will know what is right for you and will tell you the correct doses and ways of applying the remedies. Overdoses of some oils can be harmful and it's important to get the dosage right.

Bach's flower remedies

These remedies were developed by Dr Edward Bach, who practised at University College Hospital, London, in the early part of this century. He believed that people's emotional and psychological problems were at the root of much of their illness, and became critical of medical treatments which dealt only with the symptoms rather than the whole person. Influenced by homeopathy, he developed thirty-eight plant remedies from wild flowers.

The remedies are made with exactly the same ritual used by Dr Bach himself. The flower heads are placed on the surface of pure spring water and left to stand in full sunlight for three hours. The water is then strained and preserved by adding an equal volume of brandy. This is then diluted, bottled and labelled.

Dr Bach recognised that worry and fear reduce the body's resistance, making a person feel under par and making him more likely to succumb to illness, and that the worry, apprehension and irritability caused by disease hinder recovery of health and convalescence.

The remedies you choose will depend upon your state of mind. Often useful in treating people with thrush and cystitis are **crab apple**, the 'cleanser', for self-disgust and shame of ailments, and **gentian**, for despondency.

Biochemical tissue salts

Biochemics is a medical system founded by a German doctor called Schuessler in the nineteenth century. He claimed that inner harmony could be achieved through homeostatis – a balance of the body's fluid and acid–alkali levels. This balance is easily disturbed by discrepancies in mineral and trace element levels, and you can take small quantities of these salts to redress the balance.

New Era biochemical tissue salts are sold in many chemists and health shops. They are safe and easy to take and do not interact with conventional drugs.

Homeopathy

Homeopathy is the best known of the 'alternative' medicines and is growing in popularity. A distrust of relying on powerful drugs, which have side-effects and may harm the body, and a desire to be treated as a whole person and not just a body with specific symptoms are two reasons why people are increasingly turning to homeopathy.

Homeopathy is a system of medical treatment using medicine according to the principle of 'like cures like'. It was developed as a science by a German physician, Hahnemann, who noticed that quinine, which produces the same symptoms as malaria, could be used to cure it. The symptoms of a disease often show how the body is attempting to heal itself – catarrh is used to clear foreign organisms from the respiratory tract, vaginal discharges clear organisms from the reproductive tract, and so on. Homeopathy is based on this observation that substances which cause certain symptoms can also be used to cure them. However, used in conventional doses many of these substances can be toxic and extremely harmful, so in homeopathy they are increasingly diluted to render them safe. The medicines are diluted by stages in an alcohol and water solution, and vigorously mechanically shaken in between the stages in a process known as 'potentisation'.

The potency of a homeopathic remedy refers to the extent and number of times the original extract has been diluted during the preparation. For example, arnica 6c has been prepared by adding one drop of the original alcoholic extract to 99 drops of a solution of water and alcohol and shaken vigorously. One drop of this is added to another 99 drops, and so on, six times. The higher the degree of dilution, the greater the potency.

Critics of homeopathy hold that in some preparations the original substance will have been so diluted that not even one molecule of the original substance can be contained in the solution, and therefore it is impossible that it could have any effect. Homeopaths believe that during potentisation the properties of the substance being diluted are somehow imprinted into the molecules of the solution carrying it. There is no conventional scientific explanation of how this could happen, but then there are other things which modern science cannot explain.

Some scientific studies have been carried out to try to 'prove' whether homeopathy is effective or not, but since the mind is so powerful in influencing illness this is very difficult. It has been shown that 'placebos' – tablets or injections which the patient believes to contain a drug but which don't – can be highly effective in relieving even severe pain, because the patient believes it will work and relaxes. Human contact and sympathy and 'taking care of yourself' are also very powerful in relieving symptoms and pain.

Many people believe from experience and observation that homeopathy does work. It certainly cannot have any harmful consequences, so is worth trying even if you are sceptical.

Because homeopathy is holistic, the ill person's medical history, lifestyle and feelings will be taken into account. Because of this, there is no one remedy which will be useful for everyone; the remedy has to be matched to the person. In addition, the particular form the symptoms take will also affect what is prescribed. Because everyone is different, and because, particularly, cystitis can develop into a serious condition, you should always consult a professional homeopath if your symptoms are severe, or seek conventional medical treatment.

Homeopath Marie McShae writes:
I have given a symptom picture for each remedy for first cystitis and then thrush to enable you to choose the remedy which is most appropriate. The successful prescribing of homeopathic remedies relies on matching the picture of the remedy to the picture of the person who is ill. The more similar the picture, the better the chance it has of working, so the best thing to do is observe as accurately and carefully as possible.

I would suggest that you begin by using the 6 potency and move up to a 30 potency only when you are more confident. When you have decided on the remedy take one tablet and wait. When taking homeopathic remedies it is best not to eat, drink or clean your teeth ten minutes either side of taking the tablet. You should repeat the remedy if you have some response but you feel the reaction is stuck.

In general homeopathy is a gentle and effective form of medicine and can be used in the home with safety. If symptoms persist and recur, however, you may need to consult a professional homeopath. Cystitis symptoms in all instances should be carefully monitored as they can develop into a serious kidney infection and a professional should be consulted when symptoms give cause for concern.

CYSTITIS

Common symptoms of cystitis are burning pain during urination, frequent and powerful urging even though only a little urine may be passed, and cloudy or bloody urine. Pain or tenderness in the back or lower abdomen, fever and a feeling of being slightly unwell may accompany these symptoms.

There are several ways of keeping the symptoms at bay: washing carefully around the area without soap, which can be an irritant, avoiding tight clothing and in the event of an actual attack drinking a lot of water or barley water to wash out the infection. Also avoid tea, coffee, alcohol and acidic fruit.

Homeopathy can be very useful in acute flare-ups of cystitis. It can also be invaluable in treating the whole person so that a person who is susceptible can break the cycle of recurrent cystitis. Below is a list of some of the most common remedies for the acute situation.

Aconite
Indicated in the early stages, when burning sensations are first noticed.

Cantharis

There will be strong burning, cutting and stabbing pains in the lower abdomen before, during and after urination, along with a strong urge even immediately afterwards. The patient may be restless and bad-tempered.

Apis

This is similar to cantharis, though the symptoms will be less violent. The pains may be worse for heat and better for cold. The patient may be anxious and sensitive to touch. Often thirstless.

Arsenicum Album

The patient will be restless and anxious and in need of company. They will be thirsty for frequent cold drinks. Burning pains will be better for heat and warmth.

Causticum

Helpful particularly for older women. Frequent urge which can be made worse with coughing and sneezing. The person may go to the loo, fail to pass any urine, and then soon after lose urine involuntarily.

Staphysagria

Can be considered if the attack comes on after intercourse or any form of sexual abuse. It may happen after surgical intervention or painful labour. Ineffectual urging, burning and sensation as if the bladder is never emptied.

Berberis

Characterised by radiating pains which may be worse with standing or exercise. Pains in the thighs when urinating. Sensation as if urine remains after urination. Thirst alternating with thirstlessness.

THRUSH

Something like 75% of women suffer from thrush at some point, and probably 100% from itching of some sort. The most common causes of the itching and inflammation are soaps, bath salts and bubbles, talc and washing powder. It can also be caused by some contraceptives, sanitary towels and tampons, vigorous sex, tight clothing and cycling. The common symptoms of thrush are soreness, irritation, itching and a thick white discharge. There may be associated symptoms of tiredness, bloating, and a craving for sweet things, especially chocolate.

Symptoms may be kept at bay by restoring an acid environment around the vagina. This can be done by having baths with vinegar, a garlic suppository, or inserting live yogurt. Cutting down on sugar and yeast products in the diet can be helpful. Homeopathy can be useful in acute flare-ups of thrush and break the cycle of persistent or recurrent thrush.

The following remedies can be helpful if the symptom picture matches:

Borax
Discharge like egg white with the sensation as if warm water is flowing. The symptoms are worse after the period. It is almost a specific for oral thrush where you see the white patches in the mouth.

Natrium phosphoricum
Sour-smelling discharge can be creamy, or watery. Burning and itching in the genital area. Can be the result of too much sugar. Tiredness. Flatulence. A yellow-coated tongue, especially the base, is common.

Pulsatilla
Thick, burning, creamy discharge often accompanied by pain in the back and exhaustion. Itching. Worse before the

115

period. Emotionally quite tearful and wanting company. May feel better for being in the fresh air. Often thirstless.

Sepia
Discharge can be yellow or even greenish, maybe lumpy with much itching. Vagina may be dryish and painful. Worse for any sexual activity. Worse before the period. Accompanied by lower back ache and a dragging feeling. May be worn out and irritable.

Hypnotherapy
Hypnotherapy immediately conjures up an image of a man in a black suit waving a watch before your eyes and then making you do things you wouldn't normally do. Nothing could be further from the case. Hypnosis is in fact a natural state which we all experience, and is normally called dozing or daydreaming. It is not being asleep or unconscious. It is in fact self-induced and anyone who wants to can let it happen. It is experienced normally as a very relaxed, floating or pleasant feeling and you can also feel energised and alert.

Hypnotherapy means using hypnosis to work directly with the subconscious mind, channelling its resources to achieve a positive change. The subconscious mind controls our feelings and behaviour, and often a negative cycle is set up which limits us. As soon as an attack of thrush or cystitis begins, for example, we may immediately feel all the emotions of despair, depression, anger, and so on, and these negative emotions may be worse than the illness itself. Tension, stress and worry all make it harder for us to heal.

Hypnotherapy has been used very successfully to deal with pain and chronic illness. It can certainly be used to help overcome some of the negative aspects of chronic thrush and cystitis. The National School of Hypnosis and Psychotherapy and the Corporation of Advanced Hypnotherapy are members of the British Complementary Medicine Association.

Reflexology

This is a practical therapy which stimulates the body's own healing mechanism, thus creating a state of balance in the body and helping to cure illness.

In reflexology, a gentle but firm finger pressure and a special massage technique is applied to areas of the feet and lower legs which correspond to all glands, organs and parts of the body. Tensions in the body manifest themselves in the feet and hands, and the consequent blocking of energy paths results in imbalance and disease. By applying gentle pressure with the hands to relevant areas of the foot, toxins can be removed from the body and circulation improved, restoring the free flow of energy and nutrients to the body cells.

Reflexology is not a diagnostic therapy but can indicate if certain organs or glands are under pressure. It can often detect injuries which occurred years ago, and can also detect weaknesses which have not yet developed into disease.

Treatment sessions usually take between fifty and eighty minutes, and the number of treatments required varies according to the individual and the nature of the disorder. During treatment you may feel a slight discomfort on certain parts of the foot, and you may feel tired and lethargic at first, followed by a renewed sense of well-being. Reflexology can create a deep sense of relaxation, which can encourage the body's own healing processes.

Reiki

This is an ancient Japanese therapy in which hands are laid on the body to promote relaxation and natural healing. You simply relax and enjoy the warmth of the practitioner's hands over the area of pain or need. Reiki can help a variety of ailments, including cystitis and kidney complaints.

Shiatsu

Shiatsu is a Japanese therapy based on the same principles as acupuncture, in which pressure is applied to the energy lines, known as meridians. Although thumb and finger pressure is mainly used, the practitioner can also use elbows and even knees and feet.

The massage stimulates the circulation, and also the body's vital energy flow (in Japanese, Ki). Shiatsu strengthens the nervous system and helps release toxins and deep-seated tension. On a more subtle level, Shiatsu enables you to relax deeply and get in touch with your body's own healing abilities. You normally lie on a futon, and it is advisable not to eat or drink much before a treatment. A feeling of calmness and well-being usually follows a treatment, and you may well feel invigorated yet relaxed.

Visualisation

This is a technique which can help people with recurring illness or who suffer from continual pain. It is a way of focusing your mind in such a way as to help you relax and think positive thoughts which can help ease pain or make it seem less hard to bear.

Lie back and go through a relaxation exercise, relaxing all the parts of your body in turn. Then imagine that you are in some lovely place, perhaps on a tropical beach under the shade of some palm trees. Imagine the sound of the waves and the gentle breeze on your skin.

Or you could try a specific exercise for your cystitis. If you are doubled up with an attack, again, go through a relaxation technique and then imagine that your body is healing itself. Imagine, for example, the inside of your bladder and urethra turning from an inflamed red to a cool, smooth blue. Imagine the urine becoming cool and soothing, and imagine your body flushing away all the harmful things. There is some evidence that under hypnosis, parts of the body can become cooler or warmer if this is suggested to the person in a trance, and there is evidence that this suggestion can help too.

A healer often uses the same technique when they use their hands. Sally went to one when she was suffering from (another!) episode of cystitis. The healer held her hands over the bladder and said that she would first feel the area become very hot, and then cooler, and that the pain would pass off. This was exactly what happened. Sally recalls that the hot sensation was very powerful and not something she felt she could have imagined.

CHAPTER 5

Healthy Living:
How to Make
Thrush and Cystitis
a Thing of the Past

If your life has been ruined by repeated attacks of cystitis and thrush, then you need to take stock. It's not easy to make changes in the way you live. However, you may need to if you want to break out of this repeated cycle of misery and illness. You may also find this benefits you in many other ways, too.

Cystitis and thrush tend to attack when your reserves are low. Overwork, too much stress, relationship problems and emotional traumas, a poor diet and a poor working environment can all be triggers for thrush and cystitis.

THE IMPORTANCE OF DIET

It's an old truism that you are what you eat, and a great deal has been written recently about a healthy diet. There's no doubt about it, modern, processed food with colourings, preservatives and other chemicals is no good for your health. It's not just the things that are added, it's the things that are left out. Convenience food has little fibre, fewer vitamins, and can be fattening.

Much modern animal food contains hormones, antibiotics and other substances which are fed to the livestock and passed on to us. Milk contains a hormone called bovine growth hormone, and meat often contains steroids and antibiotics. It's not clear what effect this has, but one thing you can do if you eat meat is to buy organic meat and free-range chickens and to cut down on these potentially harmful additives.

In addition, avoid salty products, especially if you are prone to cystitis. Many preservatives also have to be eliminated by the kidneys and mean you produce a stronger urine, which is bad news if you are prone to cystitis.

Sugar too is bad news, both for cystitis and thrush sufferers. Eating too many sweet and sugary things overloads the bloodstream with sugar, giving you a temporary lift. The pancreas then hurriedly produces insulin to remove and store the sugar, and this often gives you a rebound reaction of feeling tired, lethargic and even faint or giddy. Cut down on sugar in drinks such as tea or coffee, avoid sugary fizzy drinks and avoid shop-bought cakes, biscuits and puddings, which are often incredibly high in sugar. If you make your own cakes and biscuits you can cut down a little on the sugar or use low sugar recipes, which can be equally delicious. Once your palate has adjusted, you may find to your surprise that you no longer enjoy such sugary things.

Eating plenty of fresh green vegetables and high-fibre foods such as beans and pulses, wholemeal bread and cereals means that you will not get constipated, and will tend to speed up the passage of waste materials through the gut, eliminating toxins from the body and thus improving your general health. Hard stools in the bowel can cause pressure during sexual intercourse which can injure the organs, causing cystitis, and there is a theory that thrush is more likely to thrive when movement of stools through the bowel is slow.

The modern diet can be short of essential minerals, too. Shortage of iron, causing anaemia, is one cause of persistent thrush. Shortage of zinc may also be another trigger.

People often believe that our modern, Western diet is better than it has ever been. Certainly the great increase in the amount of protein in our diet has meant that people today are growing much bigger and taller than in the past. But there are many harmful things about our diet, too. We tend to eat too much protein, and our bodies have to break down the proteins in order to make use of them, resulting in toxic by-products. Secondly, we eat too many fats, and these are the main cause of the very high rates of heart disease in Western countries. Thirdly, we don't eat enough fibre or roughage, causing constipation and some bowel problems. And finally, by not eating enough fresh foods, we go short of the vitamins and minerals we need.

Modern shopping habits have created problems, too. It used to be that women went out shopping almost every day in order to buy the fresh foods that they needed. Most people didn't have fridges, so meat and perishable foods had to be bought only a day or so before they were eaten. Vegetables too tended to brown and spoil quickly, so these too were bought fresh and eaten quickly.

Today people tend to shop once a week at supermarkets. The food has been bought centrally, transported and packed, and is then bought and stored at home for much of the week. Food plants are bred specially so as to have a long shelf life, rather than for nutritional value or flavour. Meats and other foods are filled with preservatives in order to last longer. 'Transgenic' tomatoes are now even being bred which won't soften when they go ripe and strawberries and other fruits are being irradiated to stop them going mouldy. Artificial flavourings and colourings are added to make up for the shortcomings of the basic produce.

I was in Russia recently and spent a week at a friend's dacha in the countryside north of Moscow. There was plenty of fresh food in the markets in Moscow if you could afford to buy it, and I was stunned at the richness in the varieties available. Almost everyone with access to an allotment or a garden grew their own food. It was absolutely delicious. The tomatoes were ripe and sweet and tasted like the tomatoes I used to eat as a child, varieties which aren't available here. The blackberries were the size of cherries. The apples, a variety I'd never seen before, were crisp and tasty and dissolved on the tongue. The sugar snap peas could be plucked from the plant and popped into your mouth instantly, and I have seldom tasted anything so delicious. Tens of different varieties of mushrooms were gathered from under the birch trees and lightly fried with butter, onions and garlic. Fresh herbs which I had never seen before were sold in little bundles. Contrary to people's expectations, I have never tasted such fresh, delicious food.

Agriculturalists may now be grateful for the large number of varieties which have survived in Russia and eastern Europe. In the future we may need these strains to make up for the shrinking genetic diversity in our own foods.

WHAT WE NEED IN OUR DIET AND WHY

The four main categories into which foods fall are carbohydrates (and sugars), proteins, fats and oils, and vitamins. All are needed for good health. It's knowing what kinds of foods contain the right amounts of these substances and knowing how much to take that is the problem.

Carbohydrates

Carbohydrates form the main source of calories in almost all diets and most staple foods are rich in it – potatoes, rice, maize, wheat. Carbohydrates are long chains of sugars. The carbohydrates are broken down into sugars first in the mouth and then the stomach. The most important sugar, on which many of the body's processes depend, is glucose. Fruits contain a sugar called fructose. Table sugar, sucrose, is a combination of fructose and sucrose linked together.

Glucose is maintained at a steady level in the blood by a number of hormones including insulin. When there is too much sugar in the diet it is then stored as a substance called glycogen in the liver.

The problem with sucrose in the diet is that it comes as 'empty' calories. When you eat naturally occurring carbohydrates, you take in vitamins, minerals and fibre, and sometimes proteins as well, as a residue of cellulose and other substances which cannot be digested and make up dietary fibre. These foods make you feel full and satisfied and provide the ingredients you need, whereas all sugar will do is give you an immediate dose of energy and tend to make you fat.

There is another problem with eating sugar as a 'quick energy' food too. When the blood sugar level goes up quickly, insulin is released to mop it up. The quicker the rise in sugar, the more insulin is released, often mopping up the sugar so quickly that the blood sugar level falls rapidly again to previous levels or lower.

If you eat complex carbohydrates, the slower process of digestion ensures that sugar is released into the bloodstream gradually, making it available to your body in a more reliable way, ensuring that you don't get the same energy peaks and troughs you will experience if you keep refuelling on sugary things.

Proteins

Proteins are essential for growth and there is a minimum amount you have to eat every day to stay healthy. Proteins are made up of long chains of amino acids. There are over twenty amino acids, some of which are essential and others not. The nine essential amino acids are those which cannot be made by the body and so must be eaten in the diet.

Non-essential amino acids can be made by the body if they are not present in the diet.

Protein is often divided into 'first class' and 'second class'. First-class proteins are those which contain significant quantities of all the amino acids. Animal meat, fish, eggs and dairy products are in this category. Second-class proteins contain some but not all amino acids, and this is the case with most vegetables. Vegetarians therefore have to take care that they eat a healthy balance of foods so that they get all the essential amino acids.

Proteins are broken down by the body into the component amino acids during digestion and then converted in the liver to the proteins which our bodies need. Proteins, unlike fats, cannot be stored by the body, so if there is too much protein in the diet this has to be broken down and metabolised, creating the substance urea, which is eliminated by the kidneys. This process puts stress on the kidneys, which is why people with kidney disease often have to have a low-protein diet to cut down the work of the kidneys.

The recommended daily allowance of protein is surprisingly small. We could get enough protein from as little as a combination of half a pint of milk, one egg, two ounces of meat, and two or three ounces of wholegrain every day.

Fats and oils

We tend to think of fats as bad, but in fact they are essential to health, being necessary for many of the body's processes. Fats provide insulation to the body and act as a store of food which the body can draw on if food is short.

Linoleic and linolenic acids are known as essential fatty acids because the body cannot make them and they have to be eaten as part of the diet. There are dozens of different fatty acids occurring naturally, and they break down into two groups, the saturated and the unsaturated fatty acids. Saturated fatty acids are found in butter, lard, meat and cocoa butter, while the unsaturated acids are liquid at room temperature, such as vegetable oils.

Some unsaturated fats are known as monounsaturated fats; these are believed to be especially good for you, and include olive oil. They are supposed to reduce cholesterol levels in the blood and thus help protect against heart disease. Fish oils are good for this too, so it's a good idea to eat oily fish such as mackerel twice a week. Polyunsaturated fats include corn and sesame oils; these seem to be less good. A lot of fried food is known to be bad for you, and certainly tends to put on the weight.

Recently there has been a controversy over many of the artificial fats found in margarines. Margarines were thought to be better for you than butter because they contained polyunsaturated fats in vegetable oils as their basis. However, in order to make them solid, they are chemically treated and form substances known as trans fatty acids, which are not known in nature. It is not clear how well the body deals with these substances and whether they are really good for your health. If you want to eat natural foods, it might be better to use a thin scrape of butter and go easy on the margarines.

If you are trying to avoid dairy products by using margarines, look carefully at the label. Many margarines use whey as their basis, with treated vegetable oils added. If you're allergic to milk, these can be just as bad as butter. There are some brands which don't contain any milk products, so check the label.

Vitamins
Everyone knows that vitamins are good for you, but most people don't know exactly why. Many vitamins are vital for processes which are carried out in the body. They also act as antioxidants, inactivating the free radicals created in the body by pollutants, cigarette smoke, radiation and chemicals in the environment.

VITAMIN A

This is found in liver, butter, cheese, margarine, eggs, carrots, tomatoes, apricots, oily fish, spinach and broccoli. Its precursor, beta carotene, is an antioxidant and is thought to help prevent cancer. Vitamin A – called retinol – is necessary for night vision and helps maintain healthy skin and mucous membranes. Early symptoms of vitamin A deficiency are night blindness and dryness of the eyes.

VITAMIN C

Found in oranges and other citrus fruits, kiwi fruit, passion fruit, blackcurrants, redcurrants, strawberries, and other fruits, and also in spinach and other dark green vegetables. It is present in particularly high levels in rosehips, and is also present in liver and kidneys. It promotes iron absorption and makes for healthy bones, teeth and gums. High doses of vitamin C are known to help protect against colds and other infections and help in wound healing. Vitamin C may have some role in preventing cancers and also seems to lower high cholesterol levels.

Lack of vitamin C produces scurvy – bleeding, swollen gums, easy bruising and a dry, scaly skin.

VITAMIN D

Found in fatty fish, cod liver oil, eggs, milk, butter and cheese. It must by law be added to margarine. The body can make vitamin D if exposed to sunlight, but in the British Isles there's precious little of that, and nowadays we are meant to avoid exposure to direct sunlight because of the risk of skin cancer. It's therefore important to take it in food.

Lack of vitamin D causes rickets – a loss of calcium to the body resulting in aches and pains in the limbs, bowed legs, and sometimes deafness.

VITAMIN B

There are twelve B group vitamins, and folic acid. They are all interlinked in terms of their action on the human body and tend to be found together in the same foodstuffs. They are found in wholegrain cereals and breads, in meat, and in peas, beans and leafy green vegetables. Some are found in high levels in nuts and seeds. It's rare to get a deficiency of one without the other, except perhaps vitamin B12.

The most important B group vitamins are:

B1, thiamine. Lack of this produces beri-beri, a Singhalese word for 'extreme weakness'.

B2, riboflavin. Dryness, cracking and peeling of the lips and red, greasy and scaly skin on the face are signs of deficiency.

B3, nicotinic acid (niacin) and **nicotinamide**. Deficiency causes pellagra, dermatitis, diarrhoea and dementia.

B6, pyridoxine. This plays an important part in protein and sugar metabolism, and in the absorption of minerals such as magnesium and zinc (see below). A scaly red rash on the face is a sign of deficiency. Large doses – above 50mg per day – can be harmful.

Vitamin B12. This B group vitamin is found only in animal products. Lack of it causes anaemia.

Folic acid. This is closely linked to vitamin B12. One of the first signs of deficiency is a sore, painful tongue. Lack of it may also cause anaemia.

VITAMIN E

This is found in vegetable oils, nuts, seeds, soya and lettuce, and there is some vitamin E in eggs and dairy produce. Like vitamin C, it can lower cholesterol levels and improve blood circulation.

Minerals

These include what are known as macrominerals, required in fairly large amounts – these are calcium, phosphorus, magnesium, sodium, potassium and chlorine – and the trace elements, which include iron, zinc, copper, manganese, iodine, chromium, selenium, molybdenum, cobalt and sulphur. Small quantities of these are needed for some essential functions.

Iron is known to be important in preventing anaemia. Iron is found in liver and kidney, egg yolk, peas and beans, cocoa and chocolate, molasses, shellfish, parsley, spinach.

Calcium is important for bones and teeth. It's found in milk, cheese, broccoli, peas and beans, leafy green vegetables, nuts, seeds, and lentils. Bran tends to bind calcium and make it difficult to absorb, so beware of adding bran to a poor diet to add fibre.

Magnesium is found in nuts, some seafoods, soya beans, whole grains, and leafy green vegetables. Tap water in hard water areas also contains magnesium. A deficiency causes extreme tiredness. Magnesium is low in processed foods and, like calcium, its absorption can be prevented by bran.

Zinc is now recognised as being a very important nutrient and a lack of it can cause infertility, especially in men, immune deficiencies, hair loss and skin conditions. Good sources are fresh oysters, ginger root, chicken, lamb, pork and beef, nuts, beef liver, egg yolk, oats, garlic, potatoes, wholewheat bread, carrots, beans, turnips, raw milk and corn.

Eating a healthy diet is very important in many ways for your physical and mental well-being. If you keep being ill, you need to look at a poor diet as a possible cause. However, there may be specific things you need to eliminate from your diet if your problem is thrush, or if it is cystitis. For both, however, it will help if you strengthen your immune system by eating certain foods and avoiding others. It's also important to remember that if you are following a strict diet, you must be sure that you are getting your daily requirement of vitamins and minerals. If you are staying on a diet for any length of time, it would be a good idea to discuss it with a dietician.

FOODS WHICH HELP YOUR IMMUNE SYSTEM

EVENING PRIMROSE OIL
This contains an essential fatty acid, gamma-linoleic acid. Evening primrose oil is marketed under a number of names, including Efamol capsules.

FISH OIL
A spoonful of the old 'cod liver oil and malt' can work wonders!

The cystitis diet
Food which can cause cystitis-like symptoms in sensitive people are spicy foods containing chilli, ordinary or cayenne pepper, monosodium glutamate (a flavour enhancer used in Chinese cooking and many processed foods), oranges, lemons, grapefruit and other citrus fruits, sugary foods, pickles, chutneys and vinegar.

The candida diet
This is the diet which has been suggested for getting rid of candida. It involves cutting out foods rich in carbohydrates or sugars, and those which contain yeasts.

You should eat vegetables, especially asparagus, broccoli, cabbage, greens, lettuce, and beans. Fish and seafood, and lean meat such as chicken and beef, and eggs are allowed. You can have unrefined vegetable oils and small amounts of butter. You can have small quantities of high-carbohydrate vegetables such as potato.

You should avoid:
Foods containing yeast:
Bread, except soda bread and unleavened bread
Pizza dough
Buns and cakes made with yeast
Marmite, Vegemite, etc.
Bovril
Oxo cubes and most stock cubes
Hydrolysed vegetable protein (look out for this in ready prepared meals)
Beer, wine, cider
Vinegar, pickles, sauerkraut
Processed and packaged foods in case they contain small quantities of any of these things
B vitamin tablets (unless 'yeast free')

Also avoid:
Anything with a high sugar content: sweets, cakes, ice cream, soft drinks and sugar-containing foods of all kinds
Dried fruit, overripe fruit, unpeeled fruit (especially if it has a 'bloom')
Commercial fruit juices
Malt
Soy sauce
Tofu
Leftover food
Blue or soft cheeses (e.g. Brie, Camembert)
Mushrooms, truffles

Some people who have tried the diet say that it works. Of course, if you've been eating a poor, mainly convenience or 'junk' food diet and switch to this you'll probably find you feel much healthier. Others say that it doesn't work and it's too difficult to stick to. Of course, you can try it, especially if you would like to lose a little weight. However, if you're busy, it's important to eat enough, and if you cut out too much carbohydrate you may find yourself feeling even more tired and drained than before.

FOOD ALLERGY

Linked to this anti-candida diet is the concept of food allergy. The idea is that people with chronic candida become allergic to certain substances in foods.

Food allergy is not a straightforward concept. Some people have an obvious and fairly prompt reaction to certain foods. If every time you eat eggs you develop a rash and vomit, you'll pretty quickly learn that you're allergic to eggs and avoid them. This reaction will occur every time you eat the substance you're allergic to, even if it's cooked and concealed in what you're eating. Common allergies of this kind are to eggs, strawberries, and certain seafoods such as lobster, shrimps etc. These allergies are easy to detect with the normal skin allergy tests.

Some diseases are caused by severe food allergies. Coeliac disease, for example, occurs when the body is allergic to gluten, a substance found in wheat and some other grains, and the body therefore doesn't digest it properly. Lactose intolerance is also one of the more common; the body cannot tolerate lactose, the sugar found in milk and milk products. The effect is the same: the body tends to eliminate all foods together with the offending ones, causing diarrhoea and severe loss of weight.

The second kind of food allergy is known as a masked or hidden food allergy. These are usually caused by foods you eat every day such as milk, wheat, or citrus fruits. These may cause problems like eczema, asthma, abdominal bloating or diarrhoea, and general malaise. You can only discover if these cause an allergic reaction by avoiding all such foods for 4–7 days and seeing if the symptoms go away. Then take a small amount of the suspected food and see if the symptoms return.

Hidden food allergies are difficult to detect and usually don't show up in the normal skin allergy tests. There is therefore controversy over them, because they can't be proven to exist. If you do think you've got a food allergy, it's worth trying eliminating the most common allergens from your diet, then slowly reintroducing them and seeing if it works.

If you are really serious, you can go on an 'exclusion diet'. The best known one is the 'pears and lamb' diet. You simply drink nothing but pure mineral water, and eat nothing but (preferably organic) lamb, pears, and wholemeal rice. You should stick to this for fourteen days. Then you begin reintroducing one food after another back into your diet every other day, and waiting to see if symptoms return. Don't overdo this, or you'll go short of essential nutrients. It's a good idea to talk to a doctor or dietician first.

You can also try avoiding foods with artificial colourings, flavourings and preservatives. These have been linked with hyperactivity in children and may affect adults too.

TAKE TIME OFF

'But I can't!' you will cry. 'I already have more work than I can cope with!' Yes, but if you get ill you will be taking time off anyway. Rushing back to work before you're fully recovered from a cystitis attack is a sure way of guaranteeing that you'll get a relapse or recurrence. If you are ill, give yourself time to recover. And then pace yourself so you don't take on too much.

Studies have shown that people who work long hours become less and less productive. It would be quite possible for a fresh, rested person to perform as much work in half a day in the office as a tired, stressed out person can achieve in ten long hours. Part-time staff often get as much done in a three-day week as full-time workers do in the full five-day

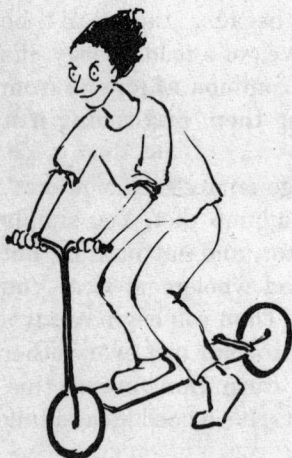

and sometimes she gets hyperactive. We think it's probably the food additives

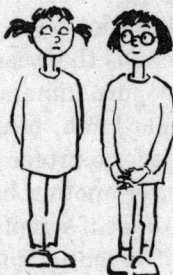

one. Having a short time to work in concentrates the mind wonderfully.

Giving yourself a day off regularly to relax, exercise, and do what you want can achieve wonders. Having your hair done, going swimming or to a sauna or Turkish bath, having a manicure – anything so long as it makes you feel good. If you are never enjoying yourself, you become depressed, and your whole being suffers.

Take a weekend away
Again, I hear you cry, 'But I can't! What about the kids? How can we afford it?'

It doesn't have to be expensive. You can go and stay with friends you haven't seen for a long time. Or you can get your mum and dad to come and stay with the children while you spend a couple of days in their house. Getting away is refreshing in itself: you can't look at your briefcase reproaching you in the corner because you haven't opened it yet, the overflowing laundry basket, or the list of letters to write and bills you have to pay.

If you really can't get away, take a break at home. Decide you're going to forget all your stressful tasks and just concentrate on enjoying yourself. One couple spent a night in a tent at the foot of their garden. They packed a picnic, took some books to read, turned the answerphone on and fell asleep under the tree listening to the rustling of the wind.

If you can, find friends to have the children overnight while you have just one whole evening and Sunday morning at home without them. It doesn't have to be much – twenty-four hours without the kids or any responsibilities can seem like a hundred years.

Hannah and Rick thought they were reaching breaking point. Rick had stresses at work, and Hannah was recovering from her third attack of cystitis. 'We packed two children off to my mum and one to a friend,' says Hannah. 'At three-thirty on Saturday they were all gone. We sat in the garden and had tea in peace and quiet. Then we thought we'd go out to a film. We walked out of the house just like that. We saw the film, had a snack in a wine bar, and came home to bed. We spent the whole of Sunday morning in bed, reading the papers, then got up and cooked a leisurely lunch. We still had time to pop out to a friend's exhibition before collecting the children at tea-time. It felt like we'd had a whole week to ourselves.'

GET REGULAR EXERCISE

Exercise is very important in keeping you fit and healthy. What's more, regular exercise has an effect on your mental state, making you feel less depressed, more alert and able to cope.

Good, brisk exercise, such as cycling, running or swimming, gets your circulation going, pumps oxygen to your brain and muscles, rids the body of toxins and gets rid of the stress and tensions you may have built up. When you are stressed your body produces a hormone, adrenalin, which makes you ready for action; for flight or fight, as they say. Unfortunately, most modern-day problems are not solved by fighting or fleeing; they require brain-power, diplomacy, or some other, sedentary skill. So the hormones go on circulating round our bodies, making us tense, anxious and angry.

Regular exercise will help burn out these emotions and restore the body to its normal state. After vigorous exercise, most people have a sense both of achievement and relaxation. You feel you've earned your rest and cup of tea, and often your brain feels more active. You feel much more able to face what lies ahead.

Unfortunately, you do need to do quite a lot of exercise regularly for it to have an effect. You need to do aerobic exercise at least three times a week for a minimum of twenty minutes to have any beneficial long-term effect. And exercise is often boring. Many people start swimming three times a week and then give up because it's so boring to swim up and down the pool fifteen or twenty times. Or going jogging gets boring and depressing once the weather gets bad.

The best thing to do is to build exercise into your day. Give yourself a bit more time for your journey into work and get out of the tube or off the bus a stop early so that you can fit in a brisk walk twice a day. Choose the most pleasant route to walk through and make it a daily routine; you'll soon find yourself strolling along at a brisk pace, thinking calmly about your day. Cycle to the shops when you need just a few items instead of taking the car. Climb the stairs at work instead of taking the lift.

Dancing is wonderful physical exercise and it's good for the spirit, too. When you have a party or friends round, don't just

136

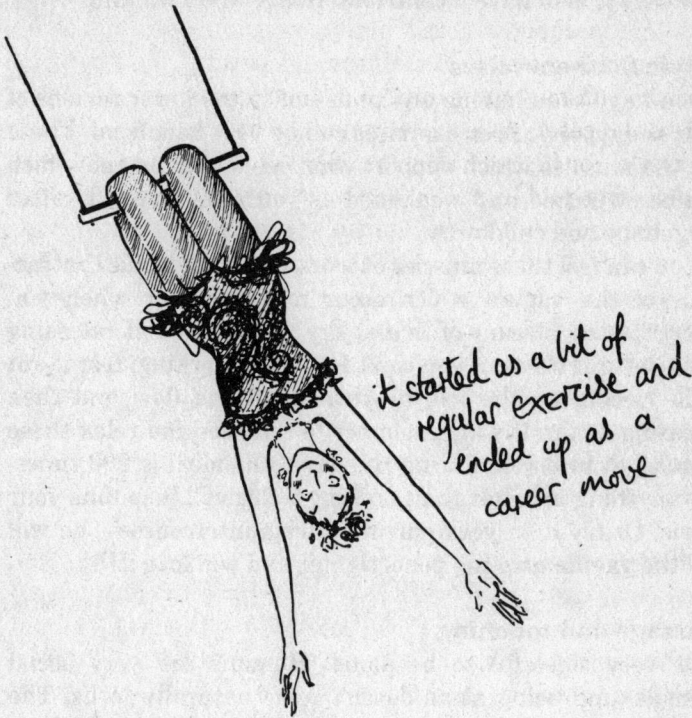

it started as a bit of regular exercise and ended up as a career move

sit around chatting and drinking, put on some good dance music, kick off your shoes and have fun. Or team up with friends and play tennis in the park once a week – it's wonderful exercise and it can be fun too. Making exercise a social occasion and doing it with friends can turn it from an act of drudgery to an enjoyable activity.

Go walking in the country at the weekends. Even some inner city walks can be beautiful – along an urban towpath, for instance, or round the city on a deserted Sunday afternoon. If you're going to see a friend, suggest you meet and go for a walk instead of having a coffee or drink – it's amazing how easy it is to have a confidential talk when walking.

Pelvic floor exercises

If you have been having any problems in the lower regions of your body, pelvic floor exercises can be very beneficial. These are the muscles which support your pelvic organs and which can be stretched and weakened as you age, especially after pregnancy and childbirth.

You can feel these muscles at work in the rhythmic contractions of the vagina which occur at orgasm or when you interrupt the stream of urine. Try clenching and releasing them several times; if you can't feel them working, test it out while peeing on the loo, by cutting off the flow and then releasing again. If you remember to contract and relax these muscles at intervals during the day – the ideal is 200 times, but anything is better than nothing – this will help tone your pelvis. Or try it on your partner during intercourse – he will feel the vagina grip the penis tighter and will love it!

Massage and touching

It is very stressful to be alone. Humans are very social animals, and being alone doesn't come naturally to us. The British tend also to be shy of touching, so that those who don't have a partner or who are in a poor relationship often find they can go for weeks at a time without even touching another human being. This is unnatural, and it's no wonder people get depressed.

If you suffer from cystitis or thrush you may also fear intimate contact with your partner; a cuddle is all very nice, but, well, one thing tends to lead to another and the last thing you want at the moment is sex. Yet research is now showing that touch stimulates the production of certain hormones and chemicals in the body, including endorphins which make you feel good and have an important role in your overall health.

Having a massage is one way of relaxing and enjoying being

touched. Done by a qualified masseur, it can make you feel wonderful. Blood circulates better, waste products are swept away from muscle cells, aches and pains caused by stress and tension can be eased. You can even do a short massage course yourself with a friend or with your partner and try it out on one another.

Flotation

One new therapy is that of flotation. A tank is filled with water containing Epsom salts and other minerals to make it buoyant, rather like the Dead Sea. The water is kept at body temperature and you lie in the water in a darkened room. You usually listen to some soothing music to begin with, and then you are left alone in the darkness and silence. The idea is that you return to a womb-like environment which is relaxing and healing both to mind and body, and some people believe it may enhance your immune system.

One side-effect of this is that flotation tanks can be an instant remedy for thrush. Working mother-of-two Cressida tried it when she felt stressed out and had been suffering from thrush on and off for some time, and said that as she lay in the water she felt a dreadful and unexpected burning sensation around her groin, which soon passed off. This one treatment cured her thrush completely and it's never come back!

RELAXATION

Many people find it hard to let go and really relax. The stresses of everyday life are too great and we move at such a fast pace that we seldom allow ourselves to come down and live at the slower pace necessary for the body to rest and recuperate.

If you learn to relax properly, even a short rest can be remarkably beneficial. You can do it anywhere – at home, even lying on the office floor – and it's completely free.

Lie on your back, arms by your sides, eyes closed. Starting at your feet, clench your muscles, then relax. Go up the legs, relaxing calves, knees, thighs, then pelvis. Tense your abdominal muscles, relax them. Then relax hands, arms, shoulders, neck, and finally, your facial muscles. Let your jaw sag if it wants to and your tongue loll in your mouth.

Think of yourself as very heavy, pressing into the floor, and the floor supporting you. Breathe slowly and perhaps more deeply than usual. Imagine, if you like, that you are in a lovely place, perhaps lying on a beach with the wind caressing your face and the rhythmic sound of the waves breaking on the shore.

Meditation

Meditation is an ideal way to reduce physical stress, to relax the mind and to help you cope with illness, grief, and other problems. Meditation is associated with religious practice, and has its place within all religions, enabling you to reach a state in which your daily preoccupations and worries fall away, and you can be 'Open to God'. You don't need to believe in God to meditate effectively or to feel the benefits, although for many people, meditating can become a religious experience.

When you meditate, your heart rate slows, blood pressure falls, respiration rates decrease and your metabolic rate is lowered. The brain wave patterns change to that of a state of alert relaxation. Meditation requires mental effort and is seldom easy for beginners, but the rewards are enormous.

In meditation, you aim to concentrate on one thing only to the exclusion of all else, thus emptying your mind of all the things that normally weigh down on it. It is fatal to try to think of emptying the mind – this will mean you inevitably feel your thoughts rushing around faster. You therefore concentrate on one thought, or an object, or your breathing, until you are aware of nothing else. You will need help to begin with, but classes are provided in many areas.

A SIMPLE MEDITATION EXERCISE

One of the most simple meditations is a Buddhist meditation called the mindfulness of breathing. You sit comfortably, cross-legged on the floor or on cushions if you can, but if you can't, and most of us are in that boat, kneeling on cushions or sitting on a comfortable straight-backed chair will help. Relax yourself, and rest your arms comfortably on your knees, preferably palms up. Go through a relaxation exercise, letting your muscles all over tense and then relax, until you feel that your body is really heavy and relaxed.

Close your eyes to cut out distractions. Breathe in and then out, quite normally, and then count one. Carry on, breathing in and then out, and count up to ten, and then count from one again. If you suddenly take a deep breath, or a very short one, note it, but don't worry.

In the second stage, you count one, then breathe in and out, anticipating the breath. In the third stage, you just breathe in and out without counting, just concentrating on each breath. In the last stage, you concentrate on the exact moment in which the breath enters your body, and on the last moment when it leaves.

It sounds easy, but it isn't. At first, lots of thoughts will crowd into your mind: did I shut the front door? Did I post the letter to so-and-so? How will I remember to ring X? Or you may find yourself remembering something you've done yesterday or wondering whether your friend has booked the house you were going to rent this summer. When this happens, don't worry or feel angry with yourself, just calmly note that this has happened and put the thoughts aside, going back to your breathing. If you lose count, don't worry, just go back to one. Don't let your own failing distract you from the state of deep relaxation which will eventually creep up on you unawares.

Those of you who are Christian may feel uneasy about what you might regard as outlandish and heathen practices, but you may know that meditative or contemplative prayer is also a part of the Christian tradition. In this kind of prayer, sit still, kneeling or on a chair, close your eyes, rest your hands palm upwards and, again, go through a simple relaxation exercise. Think about yourself being open to God. It can help to recite a simple prayer, over and over, concentrating on each word. Or you can read a short passage from the Bible, again, thinking about every word or phrase and perhaps imagining the scene in your mind. After even a short session of such prayer, you can emerge refreshed and with new energy.

All these techniques which calm and relax the body and mind will have an effect on your health. Mind and body are closely linked, and apart from helping your body build immunity, these techniques will help you deal with the depression and gloom which strikes when you are perpetually getting ill.

PSYCHOTHERAPY AND RELATIONSHIP COUNSELLING

Repeated attacks of thrush and cystitis can have a devastating effect on your personal and sexual relationships and on your self-esteem too. If a relationship is going wrong because of these attacks, or if you are not coping with your job, or if you are suffering from depression and anxiety, then psychotherapy or counselling, either individually or for you and your partner, may be just the thing you need.

It is unfortunately true that anyone can practise as a psychotherapist or counsellor with very inadequate training. You should always ask what training your counsellor or therapist has had. The British Association of Counsellors has lists of counsellors who have done a recognised course, which means they should be competent. There is also a British Association of Psychotherapy, and there are various other highly reputable organisations (see list of useful addresses on page 145).

Individually, having a session with a counsellor or therapist can give you space to talk, to air your problems and feel you are being listened to sympathetically. A good counsellor will not judge, will not advise, and will try to help put you in touch with your own feelings and make your own decisions.

If your thrush or cystitis has led to problems in your sexual relationship, and your relationship generally, as it so often does, then going for joint counselling can really help. Both partners will find it easier to express their feelings and understand one another with the counsellor acting as mediator. Grief, anger, rejection and guilt may all be involved, and if you have been unable to discuss things properly there will obviously be a great deal of underlying tension. Bringing this to the surface and expressing your feelings may lead to strong emotions, which you might be afraid to bring out alone; but with the help of an understanding therapist, these can be directed towards helping you both rather than resulting in bitter and unpleasant rows.

You can ask your GP to suggest or refer you to local sources of help or reputable therapists in your area. Alternatively, you can try Relate, which will counsel individually as well as in couples if your main problem is to do with your relationship. There are waiting lists in many areas, but it's worth getting on the list; the time may pass much quicker than you think and sometimes you may get an earlier appointment due to a cancellation.

If your sex life has taken a battering and you're finding it hard to get things going again, there are reputable sex therapists available. You can try the Institute for Psychosexual Counselling, which should be able to put you in touch with someone who can help. Most sex therapy works on the basis of going back to first principles, talking to one another and concentrating on getting pleasure out of stroking and caressing one another before progressing to full intercourse.

Of course, you may not need formal help to re-establish your sexual relationship once the trauma of repeated cystitis or thrush is in the past. This is something which, with time and goodwill on both sides, you can do yourselves. Just find time to relax together, to talk about your sexual desires and feelings as well as your fears. Take time to stroke and arouse one another before trying full intercourse, and don't be afraid to try new things. Sharing your fantasies can be wonderfully exciting, and you may find that they coincide. Don't be afraid to talk about the positions you'd prefer and how you feel most comfortable. Sex is above all a form of communication – the most intimate form there is – and talking to one another can therefore enhance it for both of you.

If your cystitis has been so bad that on occasions you feel suicidal, don't be afraid to seek immediate help. The Samaritans are always available and will give a sympathetic ear. A kind word at a crucial time can make all the difference between despair and hope.

Even if your cystitis and thrush is a thing of the past, the legacy of unhappy relationships can last for some time and overshadow your present ones. Effective counselling can help you blow away the unfinished business of the past and help you to move on to a happier and more fulfilling future.

Useful Addresses

British Complementary Medicine Association
  St Charles Hospital
  Exmoor Street
  London W10 6DZ
  (081 964 1205)

Council for Complementary and Alternative Medicine
  179 Gloucester Place
  London NW1 6DX
  (071 724 9103)

The Council for Acupuncture
  179 Gloucester Place
  London NW1 6DX
  (071 724 5756)

The British Homeopathy Association
  27a Devonshire Street
  London W1N 1RJ
  (071 935 2163)

The National Register of Hypnotherapists and Psychotherapists
  12 Cross Street
  Nelson
  Lancashire BB2 7EN
  (0282 699378)

Flotation Tank Association
    29 Sunbury Lane
    London SW11 3NP

Relate
    Herbert Grey College
    Little Church Street
    Rugby CV21 3AP
    (0788 573241)

Health Education Authority
    Hamilton House
    Mabledon Place
    London WC1A 9TY
    (071 383 3833)

The Women's Nutritional Advisory Service
    PO Box 268
    Lewes
    East Sussex BN7 2QN
    (0273 487366)

Family Planning Association
    27–35 Mortimer Street
    London W1N 7RJ
    (071 636 7866)

Women's Health Concern
    83 Earl's Court Road
    London W8 6EF
    (071 938 3932)

Women's Health
    52 Featherstone Street
    London EC1Y 8RT
    (071 251 6580)

Brook Advisory Centres (Birth Control Clinics, particularly helpful for younger people)
24-hour automated helpline
(071 617 8000)

Central office – or look in the telephone book for your local clinic
153a East Street
London SE17 2SD
(071 708 1234/1390)

The largest Sexual Health Clinic in Europe is:
Mortimer Market Centre
Capper Street
London WC1
(071 388 8880)

Further Reading

Brostoff, Dr Jonathan, and Camlin, Dr Linda, *The Complete Guide to Food Allergy and Intolerance*, London, Bloomsbury, 1992

Butterworth, Jane, *Thrush*, London, Thorsons, 1991

Crook, William G., *The Yeast Connection*, USA, Professional Books, 1986

Kilmartin, Angela, *Cystitis*, London, Thorsons, 1994

Kilmartin, Angela, *Sexual Cystitis*, London, Arrow Books, 1988

Kilmartin, Angela, *Understanding Cystitis: A complete self-help guide*, London, Arrow Books, 1989

Kilmartin, Angela, *Victims of Thrush and Cystitis*, London, Arrow Books, 1986

Index

bladder:
  bladder wash-outs 44–5
  cystoscopy 8, 33–4
bladder disorders 37, 39
  cysts 27
  irritable bladder 39
  stones 39
blood tests 31–2
blood in urine 2–3, 32
breast-feeding, thrush and
    64–5
bubble bath sensitivity 25,
    56, 61, 77
butoconizole 67

camomile 108, 109
Candida albicans 4, 57
  anti-candida diet 130–32
Canesten (clotrimazole) 67
cap (contraceptive) 23, 54–5
carbaryl 84–5
cervical cancer 91–3
  genital herpes and 87
  vaginal warts and 90
cervical erosion 97–8
cervical polyps 91
cervical smear 93, 103–4
Chemotrim (co-trimoxazole)
    41–2, 43
childbirth:
  frequency of peeing
    following 40
  urethral damage following
    37
children, cystitis in 27

chlamydia 66, 89–90
clindamycin 84
clothing aspects:
  in cystitis 25
  in thrush 61, 75–7
clotrimazole 67
co-trimoxazole 41–2, 43
coeliac disease 132
coffee 25, 47, 53
contraceptives:
  the cap and cystitis 23,
    54–5
  the cap and thrush 61
  the Pill and cervical cancer
    92
  the Pill and cystitis 55
  the Pill and thrush 59
counselling 142–4
crabs (pubic lice) 84–5
cranberry juice 46
Culpepper, Nicholas 7
Cystemme 46–7
cystitis:
  causes 19–31
  historical aspects 7
  investigations/diagnosis
    31–40
  seeking help 99–105
  signs and symptoms 2–3
  treatment 40–56
cystocele (bladder prolapse)
    37–8
cystoscopy 8, 33–4

Dalacin (clindamycin) 84

150